Review of Research in Nursing Education
Volume V

Review of Research in Nursing Education Volume V

Lois Ryan Allen, PhD, RN
Editor

National League for Nursing • New York
Pub. No. 15-2448

Copyright © 1992
National League for Nursing
350 Hudson Street, New York, NY 10014

ISBN 0-88737-542-1

This book was set in Baskerville by Publications Development. The editor and designer was Allan Graubard. Northeastern Press was the printer and binder. The cover was designed by Lillian Welsh.

Printed in the United States of America

EDITORIAL REVIEW BOARD

CONTRIBUTORS

Sharon E. Beck, EdM, MSN, RN
Assistant Professor
School of Nursing
LaSalle University
Philadelphia, Pennsylvania

Amy Bennett, MSN, RN
Nursing Instructor
Episcopal Hospital
School of Nursing
Philadelphia, Pennsylvania

Linda Dunn, DSN, RN
Assistant Professor
The University of Alabama
Capstone College of Nursing
Tuscaloosa, Alabama

Susan Gaskins, DSN, RN
Assistant Professor
The University of Alabama
Capstone College of Nursing
Tuscaloosa, Alabama

Patricia A. Haase, MS, RN
Clinical Instructor
The University of Alabama
Capstone College of Nursing
Tuscaloosa, Alabama

Joan M. Jenks, PhD, RN
Associate Professor
Department of Nursing
College of Allied Health Sciences
Thomas Jefferson University
Philadelphia, Pennsylvania

Cecile Lengacher, PhD, RN
Assistant Dean for Undergraduate Studies
College of Nursing
Health Sciences Center
University of South Florida
Tampa, Florida

Renee McLeod, MSN, RN, C, PNP
DNSc Candidate
Widener University
School of Nursing
Chester, Pennsylvania

Donna Molyneaux, MSN, RN
Assistant Professor
Graduate Nursing Program
Gwynedd Mercy College
Gwynedd Valley, Pennsylvania

Carol P. Riley, DSN, RN
Assistant Professor
The University of Alabama
Capstone College of Nursing
Tuscaloosa, Alabama

Helen J. Streubert, EdD, RN
Associate Professor
Department of Nursing
College of Allied Health Sciences
Thomas Jefferson University
Philadelphia, Pennsylvania

Cesarina M. Thompson, MS, RN
Assistant Professor of Nursing
Southern Connecticut State University
New Haven, Connecticut

Mary Lou VanCott, PhD, RN
Assistant Professor
College of Nursing
Health Sciences Center
University of South Florida
Tampa, Florida

PREFACE

The NLN Council for the Society for Research in Nursing Education is pleased to present Volume V of the Review of Research in Nursing Education series. Publication of the Review series is one way in which the CSRNE facilitates the dissemination of nursing education research findings. Each Review chapter presents an analysis of the research literature in a specific area. Beck, Bennett, McLeod, and Molyneaux discuss the complex research and measurement issues concerning critical thinking. Thompson reviews the literature describing the use of the androgogical approach with adult learners in nursing. Streubert and Jenks review the qualitative research literature in order to describe how qualitative methodology has been used to generate nursing education knowledge. Lenagacher and VanCott provide an overview of the research involving educational re-entry for the RN student. Lastly, the chapter by Haase, Riley, Dunn, and Gaskins focuses on a narrow aspect of nursing education, multiple choice examinations, but offers interesting findings that challenge the advice on test-taking strategies that faculty often give students.

Each chapter was peer reviewed by at least two members of the Editorial Board. As Editor of this volume, I want to express my sincere appreciation to the members of the Editorial Board for their time, effort, and expertise in critiquing manuscripts.

I will continue as Editor for Volume VI and invite all inquires, letters of interest, or outlines for chapter submissions.

Lois Ryan Allen, PhD, RN
Associate Professor
Widener University
School of Nursing
Chester, PA 19013

CONTENTS

Editorial Review Board
Contributors
Preface

1. **Review of Research on Critical Thinking in
    Nursing Education**   1
    *Sharon E. Beck, Amy Bennett, Renee McLeod, and
    Donna Molyneaux*

2. **Nontraditional Students in Higher Education: A
    Review of the Literature and Implications for
    Nursing Education**   31
    Cesarina M. Thompson

3. **Qualitative Research in Nursing Education**   45
    Helen J. Streubert and Joan M. Jenks

4. **Nursing Research Related to Educational Re-Entry
    for the Registered Nurse**   75
    Cecile Lengacher and Mary Lou VanCott

5. **A Review of Literature on Changing Answers on
    Multiple-Choice Examinations**   107
    *Patricia A. Haase, Carol P. Riley, Linda Dunn, and
    Susan Gaskins*

Chapter One

REVIEW OF RESEARCH ON CRITICAL THINKING IN NURSING EDUCATION

Sharon E. Beck, EdM, MSN, RN
Amy Bennett, MSN, RN
Renee McLeod, MSN, RN
Donna Molyneaux, MSN, RN

INTRODUCTION

Health care today has many complex problems that cannot be solved unless significant conceptual shifts are made by the providers of that health care. Most health care problems are multidimensional as well as multi-system and involve values and priorities that demand sympathetic consideration of all points of view and an interdisciplinary approach. Reductive thinking within the discipline of nursing does not equip future nurses with the ability to solve such problems. How to teach nursing students to make appropriate clinical decisions and to make the conceptual shifts that will be necessary to keep nursing in the forefront of health care delivery in the future is one of the major dilemmas facing nursing educators today.

Paul (1990) has stated that "instructional practice in most academic institutions around the world presupposes a didactic theory of knowledge, learning and literacy, ill-suited to the development of critical minds and literate persons. After a superficial exposure to reading, writing, and arithmetic, schooling is typically fragmented into more or less technical domains each with a large vocabulary and an extensive content or propositional base (p. 20)." Nursing education today is no exception to this observation.

Nursing education today is still basically lecture and drill despite the current curriculum revolution. Shallow and speedy coverage of a topic is often followed by content-specific testing. Synthesis of the material from different courses and application to

1

the "real world of practice in the clinical area is seen as the personal responsibility of the student and is not routinely tested."

The didactic method of instruction does not allow students to learn how to gather, analyze, synthesize, and assess information. These are skills that are critical to the practice of nursing. Nursing students frequently do not learn how to analyze the diverse logics of questions and problems that will face them in the clinical area and therefore they may be unable to function in the clinical area. These critical thinking and creative problem solving skills are necessary components of clinical judgment. Miller and Malcolm (1990) believe that nurses need critical thinking skills in order to practice as safe competent practitioners. Paul (1990) believes that critical thinking ability is necessary for the advancement of knowledge since it allows students to explain and understand the basis for their beliefs and the decisions that are made based on those beliefs.

Kurfiss (1988) sees critical thinking as an investigation whose purpose is to explore or discover a situation, phenomenon, question or problem in order to arrive at a hypothesis or make conclusions about the hypothesis. The conclusion integrates all available information and can therefore be justified, and supportive arguments can be developed. As Kurfiss states, "in critical thinking, all assumptions are open to question, divergent views are aggressively sought and the inquiry is not biased in favor of a particular outcome" (p. 2).

Although knowledge enhances a person's potential, the inability to reflect critically and rationally about ideas hampers that potential. Critical inquiry, as a necessary part of critical thinking, leads students to a capacity to draw conclusions and make decisions with confidence. They can analyze alternatives and such analysis enables them to argue and defend their ideas and conclusions with confidence.

Kurfiss (1988) proposes that faculty must take an active role to assist students to "cultivate" thinking skills. Effort must be made to stimulate critical thinking throughout the curriculum. Paul (1990) believes that the only way this can happen is for courses to be conducted using Socratic instruction, in which students are allowed to discuss and develop their thinking and ideas by making them explicit. According to Pardue (1987) "the key component of nursing practice is the nurse's ability to process information and to make decisions" (p. 354). The Socratic method of instruction could increase the students' ability to make decisions.

An examination of articles written and research conducted pertinent to critical thinking in nursing reveals information that is grouped into three different but related areas: (1) creative problem solving; (2) clinical judgment skills; and (3) critical thinking. In a recent review of studies of critical thinking and clinical judgment in nursing, Kintgen-Andrews (1991) found no support for a relationship between critical thinking ability and clinical judgment. Critical thinking may be an essential skill for problem solving and clinical judgment, but even if it is a component of problem solving and clinical judgment, it is not identical to them. For the purposes of this paper, the relationship between nursing education and critical thinking as a concept distinct from clinical judgment will be explored within the framework of nursing research.

HISTORICAL BACKGROUND

A brief overview of some of the historical influences originating in Western philosophy on the current views of critical thinking enhances the understanding of this concept. These theories of critical thinking demonstrate the basic views that have been influential in the development of critical thinking as it is known today.

Greek Philosophers

The idea of contemplating a problem for its own sake and not only for its relation to human needs was first introduced by the Greeks. For Socrates, "the uninquiring life is not the life for man" (Furedy & Furedy, 1985, p. 54). Socrates embraced and improved the questioning critical attitude. He proposed that all traditions and assumptions were open to critical examination. For Socrates, purposefully thinking about an idea or an assumption and weighing logical arguments against one another helps to clarify ideas and positions (Anderson, 1961).

Plato was a student of Socrates and the Socratic influences on his beliefs about thinking are apparent. According to Aune (1967), in Platonism "thinking is either a dialogue in the soul involving mental words that he refers to as 'forms' . . . or a spiritual activity of inspecting or recollecting 'forms' and discerning their natures and interrelations" (p. 101). Plato believed that education not only provides information, but should help students to question, examine and reflect upon ideas and values.

Aristotle, in the *Nicomachean Ethics* (translated by Oswald, 1962), believed that thinking is an act of the intellect. Clarification occurs the more we think about something and results in knowledge. Aristotle suggested that critical thinking involves abstract thinking and logical thinking. He connected thinking and values, and developed the idea that moral reasoning is linked to critical thinking.

Modern Influences

A major influence in modern concepts of critical thinking is John Dewey. Dewey (1916) proposed that thinking begins in an ambiguous situation that causes a dilemma and proposes alternatives. "Thinking includes . . . the sense of a problem, the observation of conditions, formation and rationale, elaboration of a suggested conclusion, and the active experimental testing" (p. 158). If certain results or consequences occur, validity can be established. Dewey suggested that the reflective process guides critical thinking and involves thorough assessment and scrutiny and the drawing of a conclusion. This decision making and assessment of information contributes to judgment. Critical thinking involves suspension of judgment and healthy skepticism. In order to promote critical thinking, education should follow the reflective process. Educators should capitalize on students' interests and experiences to make the learning process real. The aim of education, for Dewey, is for students to develop intellectually as well as morally.

Another influential thinker in the area of critical thinking is Edward Glaser. Glaser (1941) proposed three components to critical thinking: (1) an attitude of being disposed to consider problems and subjects within one's experiences; (2) knowledge of the methods of logical inquiry and reasoning; and (3) skill in applying these methods (pp. 5–6). Glaser considered critical thinking as a general ability that can be measured independent of content or knowledge of subject.

William Perry (1970), a cognitive theorist, has also been influential in our understanding of the thinking process. He studied students' ways of perceiving knowledge, truth, and authority. He believes that students' cognitive growth progresses through the stages of dualism, multiplicity, relativism and commitment. In dualism, the individual has difficulty with tasks requiring recognition of conflicting viewpoints. Authorities (i.e., teachers) have the right answer for every problem. In multiplicity, the students begin to see that there are conflicting opinions and that this is a necessary part of knowledge. In the stage of relativism, diversity of opinions and values are connected by the student to the context. Recognition of knowledge is relative and will develop from the student's own experiences and judgment. In the stage of commitment, an individual makes an initial commitment, accepts the implications of a pluralistic world and experiences the implications of the commitment and its responsibilities. Progression through these stages leads to the student's recognition of the "indeterminacy of knowledge and with that, a recognition of personal responsibility for making judgments and commitments in a relativistic world" (Kurfiss, 1988, p. 11). The process of making these judgments and commitments involves the use of critical thinking skills.

DEFINING THE CONCEPT OF CRITICAL THINKING

There is a paucity of relevant research on critical thinking in nursing education. One reason is the lack of an agreed-upon general definition of critical thinking for education in nursing. Proposed definitions reflect goals of critical thinking, the process, the methodology, critical attributes, or the scope of critical thinking. The concept continues to have different meanings for different people. A review of different perspectives of the meaning of the concept is therefore necessary in order to look at the relevant research.

Watson and Glaser (1964) claim critical thinking is an attitude of being disposed to consider in a thoughtful way the problems and subjects that come within the range of one's experience. It also involves knowledge of the methods of logical inquiry and reasoning as well as skill in applying these methods. Halpern (1984) adds that critical thinking is directed thinking that is purposeful and goal directed. It occurs in solving problems and drawing inferences as well as in making decisions. Critical thinking is contrasted with non-directed thinking, which is routine and underlies our daily habits. Facione (1984) further claims that critical thinking is something that every intelligent person engages in. He assumes that reasoning and critical thinking are not coextensive. "Reasoning is a broader concept; all critical thinking is good reasoning, but not all good reasoning is critical thinking" (p. 255). Facione proposes that an operational definition is that "critical thinking is the development and evaluation of arguments" (p. 257).

Norris (1985) believes that "having a critical spirit is as important as thinking critically. The critical spirit requires one to think critically about all aspects of life, to think critically about one's own thinking and to act on the basis of what one has considered when using critical thinking skills" (p. 44). Finally, Ennis (1985) believes that critical thinking is reflective. He defines critical thinking as "a reflective and reasonable thinking that is focused on deciding what to believe or do" (p. 45). Ennis claims three dimensions of critical thinking: "(1) logical dimensions; (2) critical dimensions; and (3) pragmatic dimensions" (p. 117). The logical dimension covers knowing the meaning of words and statements in a particular domain as well as the ability to use logical operations. The critical dimension involves knowledge of the criteria for judging statements. The pragmatic dimension deals with the appropriateness and acceptability of the decisions and the judgments. Critical thinking, according to Ennis (1989), involves subject specificity—that is, adequate knowledge of a particular subject is necessary for critical thinking to occur. Unlike Glaser, Ennis does not believe critical thinking is context free.

Instruments Used to Measure Critical Thinking

The concept of critical thinking has different meanings among researchers and educators. Because of this factor, research must rely on adequate operational specification. One tool widely utilized to measure critical thinking is the Watson-Glaser Critical Thinking Appraisal Test (1980), and another is the Cornell Test of Critical Thinking developed by Ennis and Millman (1985). The KneWi instrument (Widick, 1975), also used by some researchers, measures Perry's stages of cognitive development.

The Watson-Glaser Critical Thinking Appraisal (WGCTA) (1980), the most widely used critical thinking test in nursing, is designed to measure critical thinking as a general ability. It was designed to measure ability to recognize assumptions and inferences and to evaluate arguments and conclusions. This 80 item standardized tool contains five subject areas and yields one total score. There are two formats available, A and B. Having these two formats is useful to the researcher using a pretest, posttest procedure. The five subject areas are: inference, recognition of assumptions, deductions, interpretation and evaluation of arguments.

The WGCTA tests logical inquiry and reasoning. Scores are reported as the number of correct items. Reliability was confirmed by internal consistency determined by the split-half method. Construct validity was established by the use of the test in instructional settings designed to improve critical thinking and by comparison with other mental ability and comprehension tests. The test is content free and requires no specific knowledge of any discipline specific content. Therefore the test can be utilized as a measure of general critical thinking ability.

McMillan (1987) reviewed studies of critical thinking on college students from 1951 to 1983, many of which used the WGCTA to measure critical thinking. Two studies examined the effects of a program or a general college effect on students' critical thinking; in both studies it was difficult to separate the effects of college from maturation or the effects of the program from out of class experiences. Four studies examined the effects of specific courses or programs on critical thinking; two found no significant differences between the treatment and control groups and two had mixed results. Five studies of the effects of instructional variables on critical thinking found no significant differences between the treatment and control groups; two more studies of instructional variables had mixed results; and another found the control group showed significantly more increase in critical thinking ability than the experimental group.

McMillan (1987) suggests several reasons why the research using the WGCTA test produced such ambiguous results. One is that the WGCTA is not a sensitive enough measure to show changes in critical thinking ability over such a short time as a course or a semester. Another is that the WGCTA was developed to evaluate the ability to think critically about situations in daily life, and thus it may not be a good instrument for measuring changes in the context of a specific course or class. Alternatively, McMillan suggests that the treatments being studied were not strong enough to produce measurable changes.

Ennis and Millman (1985) have developed the Cornell Test of Critical Thinking Ability, which is used for measuring critical thinking. One form of the test is for the college-level student and evaluates reasoning (inductive or deductive), and the ability to identify assumptions, fallacies, definitions, and predictions. This test was not used in any of the nursing research reviewed.

Widick (1975) redefined Knefelkamp's cognitive development instrument which is now referred to as KneWi. This measure consists of two essay questions that enable students to share their thinking and processing of a subject. These essays measure dualism, relativism and commitment. Students' placement on the Perry scale is determined by essays scored by trained raters. The KneWi instrument is used in only one of the research studies reviewed.

NURSING EDUCATION RESEARCH ON CRITICAL THINKING

The following studies investigated the relationship of critical thinking to a variety of factors. Some studies examined correlations between critical thinking and other measures of success in nursing education. Some studies attempted to investigate the effects of nursing education on critical thinking abilities. Other studies examined the relationships between critical thinking and clinical decision making and moral reasoning in nursing students and in practicing nurses from professional and technical nursing education programs. Generalizations should be made from these studies with caution, as the samples studied were not selected randomly; most were convenience samples of volunteers. In addition, no studies were identified which replicated previous research.

Critical Thinking as a Correlate of Success in Nursing

Tiessen (1987) studied which selected variables correlated most strongly with critical thinking abilities of students in a four year BSN program. Eight independent variables were studied: (1) SAT verbal scores (SAT V); (2) SAT quantitative scores (SAT M); (3) grade point average (GPA); (4) age; (5) total number of college credit hours in the natural sciences (NSCI); (6) total number of college credit hours in the behavioral/social sciences; (7) total number of college credit hours in arts and humanities (AHUM); and (8) total number of college credit hours in professional nursing courses. Critical thinking was measured using the Watson-Glaser Critical Thinking Appraisal (WGCTA). Tiessen's sample was a convenience sample of 150 volunteer students from a BSN program: 41 freshmen, 37 sophomores, 38 juniors, and 34 seniors. These volunteers constituted about one quarter of the students in the program.

Tiessen found correlations which were significant at the p < .01 level for SAT M (.38), SAT V (.33), GPA (.32), and AHUM (.30). Using multiple regression, she found a correlation between critical thinking, SAT M, AHUM, and GPA of .49, which accounted for 24% of the variance in critical thinking (SAT M 14%, AHUM 8% and GPA 2%). The other variables were intercorrelated with SAT M, AHUM and GPA. Tiessen reported that math ability correlated most strongly with critical thinking. Tiessen believed math ability was a critical ability for nursing practice, and therefore was a good predictor of success in a nursing program and a valid criterion for admission. Courses in the arts and humanities were seen as promoting inquiry and problem solving, but they were also good indicators of the amount of time spent in this particular program. Thus, the correlation between critical thinking abilities and credit hours in the arts and humanities may reflect a general college effect rather than a program effect.

Bauwens and Gerhard (1987) also investigated predictors of success in a BSN program. The two independent variables studied were critical thinking, as measured by the WGCTA during the first week of enrollment in the nursing program, and the university GPA prior to admission to the nursing program (pre-nursing GPA). Four dependent variables were studied: the WGCTA score shortly before graduation, GPA and nursing cumulative average at graduation and the National Counsel Licensing Examination (NCLEX-RN score). GPA at graduation was dropped from the analysis due to high correlations with the pre-nursing GPA and the nursing cumulative average. The sample studied was a convenience sample of 159 volunteer students of an upper division BSN program (from a total population of 177 graduates).

Using correlation statistics and multiple regression, Bauwens and Gerhard found that the pre-nursing GPA was strongly correlated with the nursing cumulative average (.62 with p < .005), and that the entry WGCTA score accounted for 28% of the variance in the graduation WGCTA score. Pre-nursing GPA and the entry WGCTA scores accounted for 22% of the variance in NCLEX scores (p < .01). These findings suggest that critical thinking is a good predictor of success in nursing and that the WGCTA is a useful pre-admission screening tool.

Bauwens and Gerhard (1987) found no significant differences between entry and graduation WGCTA scores. This result implies that nursing education does not produce gains in critical thinking as measured by the WGCTA. Bauwens and Gerhard

Table 1. Studies of Critical Thinking Reviewed

Problem	Design	Instruments	Subjects	Results
Tiessen, 1987 What variables correlate most strongly with critical thinking ability?	Correlational	WGCTA	Convenience sample of 150 volunteer students from a 4-year BSN program	Critical thinking showed positive correlation with SAT math scores, college credit hours in the arts and humanities, and GPA
Bauwens & Gerhard, 1987 What are early predictors of success in a BSN program?	Correlational	WGCTA	Convenience sample of 159 volunteer students from an upper division BSN program	Entry critical thinking scores and pre-nursing GPA showed positive correlation with NCLEX scores. There were no significant differences between entry and graduation critical thinking scores.
Gross, Takazawa, & Rose, 1987 What is the usefulness of critical thinking and NLN pre-admission exam scores as selection criteria for admission? Also, what is the effect of nursing education on critical thinking ability?	Correlational Pretest/posttest with no control group	WGCTA	Convenience sample of 60 AD and 60 upper division BSN students	Entry critical thinking scores showed positive correlations with NLN total and verbal scores and with the BSN students' GPAs; no significant correlations with the math NLN, nor with the AD students' GPAs, nor with the NCLEX scores of either AD or BSN students. There were significant increases in critical thinking scores from entry to graduation for both groups.
Valiga, 1983 What are the differences in cognitive development among freshmen, sophomore, junior and senior	Comparative Pretest/posttest with no control group	Kne-Wi (Perry scheme)	Random selection of BSN students, then 123 volunteers from that group;	On both pretest and posttest, seniors scored significantly higher than freshmen. There were no significant changes

Author / Question	Design	Instrument	Sample	Findings
nursing students? Also, what changes in cognitive development occur in baccalaureate nursing students over an academic year?			approximately equal number of freshmen, sophomores, juniors and seniors	from pretest to posttest for any group.
Berger, 1984 What is the relationship of between critical thinking and GPA? What are the differences between the critical thinking abilities of sophomore BSN students and liberal arts freshmen and seniors? Are there any changes in critical thinking abilities of BSN students from their sophomore to their senior years?	Correlational Comparative Pretest/posttest with no control group	WGCTA	137 BSN students (no information given on method of selection)	There was no significant correlation between critical thinking and GPA. Sophomore nursing students had significantly higher critical thinking scores than freshman or senior liberal arts students. There was a significant increase in the nursing students' critical thinking scores from their sophomore to their senior year.
Sullivan, 1987 What are the relationships among critical thinking, creativity, clinical performance and academic performance? Does critical thinking improve during a two year RN to BSN program?	Correlational Pretest/posttest with no control	WGCTA Torrence test of Creative Thinking Slater-Stewart Evaluation of Nursing Scale	Intact sample of 51 students in an RN to BSN program	There were positive correlations between individual students' entry and exit critical thinking scores, and between entry and exit GPA and creativity measures. There was no change in the average critical thinking scores from entry to exit.
Fleeger, 1987 What are the relationships among critical thinking, moral reasoning, and	Correlational Comparative	WGCTA Rest's Defining Issues Test	Purposive cross-sectional sample: 91 students from the upper three	There was a weak but positive relationship between critical thinking and moral reasoning.

Table 1. (*Continued*)

Problem	Design	Instruments	Subjects	Results
aptitude and achievement? What is the effect of BSN education on critical thinking and moral reasoning?		SATs	levels of a 5 year BSN program, 41 Level I, 23 Level II, & 27 Level III	There were significant positive relationships between aptitude and achievement and critical thinking and moral reasoning. There were no significant differences among the three Levels in critical thinking or moral reasoning.
Lynch, 1988 What is the relationship between critical thinking and age and SATs? How do the critical thinking abilities of generic BSN students compare with those of AD students?	Correlational Comparative	WGCTA	Convenience sample of 87 AD and 74 BSN students	There was no correlation between critical thinking and age; there was a positive correlation between critical thinking and SATs. The critical thinking abilities of the BSN students were significantly higher than those of the Ad students.
Kintgen-Andrews, 1988 How do critical thinking abilities and their development differ among career ladder PN students, AD students, pre-health science freshmen and sophomore BSN students?	Comparative Pretest/posttest	WGCTA	Intact samples of 55 PN students and 55 second year AD students, and convenience volunteer samples of 38 pre-health science freshmen and 29 sophomore BSN students	There were no significant differences in critical thinking abilities between the PN students and the pre-health science freshmen. The BSN sophomores had significantly higher critical thinking abilities than the AD students. There were no significant increases in critical thinking abilities in any group over an academic year.

Study / Research Question	Design	Instrument	Sample	Findings
Brooks & Shepherd, 1990 What is the relationship between critical thinking and clinical decision-making? How do the critical thinking and clinical decision-making abilities of students in diploma, AD, and RN completion and generic BSN programs differ?	Correlational Comparative	WGCTA Gover's Nursing Performance Simulation Instrument	Convenience sample of volunteer students: 50 each from diploma, AD, RN, and generic BSN programs	There was a weak but significant relationship between critical thinking and clinical decision-making abilities in all programs. The critical thinking abilities of both types of BSN students were significantly higher than those of the diploma or AD students; there was no significant difference between the critical thinking abilities of the RN and generic BSN students. The clinical decision-making abilities of the RN students were significantly higher than those of all other students.
Pardue, 1987 What are the differences in critical thinking and clinical decision-making among the graduates of diploma, AD, BSN and MSN programs?	Comparative	WGCTA Researcher-developed clinical decision-making tool	Stratified random sample of RNs, then 121 volunteers from that group; approximately equal numbers from each type of program	The critical thinking abilities of the BSN and MSN graduates were significantly higher than those of the diploma and AD graduates. There were no significant differences among any of the groups in clinical decision-making abilities
Matthews & Gaul, 1979 What is the relationship between critical thinking ability and the ability to derive nursing diagnoses? How do these abilities differ between senior BSN students and graduate students?	Correlational Comparative	WGCTA Researcher-developed case study to evaluate nursing diagnosis ability	Purposive sample of 22 BSN students and 26 graduate students	There was no correlation between critical thinking ability and ability to derive nursing diagnoses. There were no significant differences between the groups in critical thinking abilities; however, the graduate students were significantly better able to identify nursing diagnoses than the BSN students.

Table 1. (*Continued*)

Problem	Design	Instruments	Subjects	Results
Ketefian, 1981 What are the relationships among critical thinking, moral judgment and level of educational preparation? How do the moral judgment levels of professional and technical nurses differ?	Correlational Comparative	WGCTA REST's Defining Issues Test	Convenience sample of volunteer RNs, 36 technical level and 43 professional level	There was a significant positive relationship between critical thinking and moral judgment, and critical thinking and level of educational preparation together were significantly correlated with moral judgment. The moral judgment levels of professional nurses were significantly higher than those of technical nurses.

suggest that this finding may reflect the WGCTA emphasis on logical thinking rather than on the problem solving process. However, any interpretation of this result should be made with caution, because only 53 students from the sample took the WGCTA just before graduation.

Gross, Takazawa, and Rose (1987) examined the relationships among the WGCTA, age, years of previous higher education and National League for Nursing pre-admission exam scores (verbal, math, and science) as selection criteria for admission. They also studied the impact of nursing education on students' ability to think critically using a pretest/posttest design with no control group. Critical thinking was measured by the WGCTA at entry into the program and at exit. The group studied was a convenience sample of 120 students: 60 AD and 60 upper division BSN students. Because the school was in the process of phasing out the generic upper division BSN program and replacing it with an articulated AD/BSN program, both groups of students were recruited from the same pool. There was considerable attrition in the sample; 22 AD and 4 BSN students dropped out and 1 AD and 22 BSN students did not retake the WGCTA at the end of the program.

For both the AD and the BSN groups, Gross, Takazawa, and Rose (1987) found no significant correlations between admission WGCTA scores and age or years of previous higher education. They did find significant correlations between admission WGCTA scores and the total and verbal NLN scores (.28 for the total and .37 for the verbal, p < .05), but unlike Tiessen, they found no significant correlations between admission WGCTA scores and the math or science NLN scores. For the BSN students only, there was a significant correlation between the admission WGCTA scores and the cumulative GPA (.32, p < .05); there was no significant correlation between the admission WGCTA scores and the NCLEX scores for either group. According to Gross, Takazawa, and Rose, the WGCTA appeared to be a useful predictor of success in nursing education.

For both the AD and the BSN students for whom entry and exit WGCTA scores were available, Gross, Takazawa, and Rose (1987) found highly significant improvements in the mean scores from entry to exit (p < .000). Due to the nearly 30% attrition rate from the sample, this result should be viewed with caution. Furthermore, with no control group, maturation and the general college effect cannot be ruled out as alternative explanations for these results.

Tiessen (1987), Bauwens and Gerhard (1987), and Gross, Taka-zawa, and Rose (1987) studied the correlations between critical thinking and other variables as predictors, which can be selected for, not as variables which can be manipulated. Although critical thinking was found to be a good predictor of success in all three studies, these correlational studies give little indication of whether or how nursing programs can improve students' critical thinking abilities. Bauwens and Gerhard, and Gross, Takazawa, and Rose did examine changes in critical thinking from entry to exit; Bauwens and Gerhard found no significant changes, and Gross, Takazawa, and Rose found highly significant changes. However, both studies studied small samples for this particular phenom-enon. The following studies specifically examined the effects of nursing education on critical thinking.

Effects of Nursing Education on Critical Thinking Ability

Valiga (1983) investigated the cognitive development of nursing students among freshmen, sophomores, juniors, and seniors and the changes that occurred over an academic year using a pretest/posttest design with no control group. Valiga defines cognitive development as the ability to structure and organize knowledge and experience, to deal with conflicting information and diversity of interpretation of data, and to make independent decisions. This definition is similar to most definitions of critical thinking. Valiga measured cognitive development early in the fall and late in the spring, using the KneWi instrument with 123 students from three BSN programs. Students were selected at random and invited to participate in the study, and the final group consisted of volun-teers. There were 29 freshmen, 27 sophomores, 34 juniors, and 33 seniors. Valiga controlled for an instrumentation threat to validity by having the KneWi results from all the groups, both pretests and posttests, scored at once by a trained rater who was blind to the student levels and to the pre- or posttest status of each test.

Most of the students' scores, and all of the means, fell into the dualism category of Perry's stages of cognitive development. No scores were higher than the relativism category. Analysis revealed that on the pretests, freshman scores were significantly lower than sophomore and senior scores ($p < .01$). On the posttests freshman scores were significantly lower than senior scores ($p < .01$). No other group comparisons were significant. There were no signifi-cant changes in the scores from fall to the spring. Valiga's study provides partial support for the position that nursing education improves cognitive development, but since the change does not occur over the span of the academic year, the differences among the classes could be random rather than developmental. Additionally, because the KneWi instrument has a different conceptual basis from Watson and Glaser, the KneWi results are not directly comparable to the more commonly used WGCTA tool.

Berger (1984) compared the critical thinking abilities of sophomore nursing students in a BSN program to those of liberal arts freshmen and seniors, studied changes in the critical thinking scores of the nursing students from their sophomore to their senior year using a pretest/posttest design with no control group, and examined the relationship of critical thinking scores to GPA. Critical thinking was measured using the WGCTA. The group studied was 137 students in a BSN program; no information was given on how the sample was selected. Berger found that the sophomore nursing students scored significantly higher in critical thinking than either freshman or senior liberal arts students. There was a significant increase in the nursing students' scores from their sophomore scores to their senior scores. There was no significant relationship between the nursing students' critical thinking scores and the GPA. (The level of significance for these statistics was not given.) This study supports the position that nursing education improves critical thinking ability, but the statistical information given is inadequate to judge whether the results are generalizable. Berger defines the study as descriptive and suggests further research.

Sullivan (1987) investigated whether critical thinking improved during enrollment in a two year RN to BSN nursing program, using a pretest/posttest design with no control group. Sullivan also investigated the relationship between critical thinking, creativity, clinical performance and academic performance. Critical thinking was measured using the WGCTA, creativity using the Torrence Test of Creative Thinking (cited in Sullivan, 1987) and clinical performance using the Slater-Stewart Evaluation of Nursing Scale (cited in Sullivan, 1987). All three instruments were administered at the beginning and end of the BSN program. Academic performance was measured using the students' entry and exit GPAs. The group studied was an intact sample of 51 RN students in the RN to BSN program.

The results showed that the group's average WGCTA scores were the same at entry and exit. Significant positive correlations (p < .05) were found between individual students on the entry and exit WGCTA scores and between the entry and exit GPA and the creativity measures. Sullivan's study does not support the position that baccalaureate nursing education improves critical thinking abilities. One explanation is that the students were only in the program for two years, but Gross, Takazawa, and Rose (1987) found significant changes in two years of an AD program. Another consideration in Sullivan's study is that it is based on a group of RN baccalaureate completion students rather than generic BSN students. There is no information available to compare the RN to BSN students' entry critical thinking skills with the entry critical thinking skills of generic BSN students. The critical thinking skills of the RN to BSN students may already be high enough that BSN education has no significant effect.

Fleeger (1987) studied the effect of baccalaureate nursing education on critical thinking as part of a larger study. Using the WGCTA, she compared the critical thinking abilities of students in the upper three years of a five year BSN program. The sample consisted of three groups identified using a purposive cross-sectional method: 41 Level I students tested at the beginning of their first clinical course, 23 students in the first semester of Level II, and 27 students tested during the first and last semesters of Level III. The analysis revealed no significant differences among the groups in critical thinking abilities. This study did not support the position that baccalaureate nursing education improved critical thinking abilities.

Gross, Takazawa, and Rose (1987), Valiga (1983), Berger (1984), and Sullivan (1987) each used a pretest/posttest design with no control group to study changes in critical thinking from entry into a nursing program to exit. Without a control group, there is no way to control for the internal threats of history and maturation to the validity of these studies. It is not possible to rule out the general effects of the college experience and of maturation to explain the increases in critical thinking of the students from entry to exit in these studies.

Effects of Different Types of Nursing Programs on Critical Thinking

Lynch (1988) took a different approach to investigate the effect of nursing education on critical thinking abilities. She studied the relationship between the level of nursing education and critical thinking by comparing the critical thinking abilities of graduating generic BSN students and graduating AD nursing students. She also investigated the possibility of covariance of students' ages and SAT scores with critical thinking. The WGCTA was used to measure critical thinking. Age was obtained from a demographics questionnaire and SAT scores from students' records. The convenience sample of volunteers consisted of 87 AD students from four programs and 74 BSN students from three programs.

The results indicated that the mean WGCTA score for the BSN students was significantly higher than the mean for the AD students (p < .001). There was no significant correlation between the WGCTA scores and the students' ages. Multiple regression analysis did find a significant correlation between the SAT scores and WGCTA scores; in fact, when the group whose SAT scores fell in the semi-interquartile range (25th through 75th percentile) was examined, there was no significant difference between the AD and BSN groups. This implies that the difference between the two groups may be in the selection into the program, and not in the educational program itself. However, the validity of this interpretation is weakened by the small size of the AD group which fell into the semi-interquartile range on the SATs (n = 18).

Kintgen-Andrews (1988) also compared the critical thinking abilities of students in different levels of nursing education, and the effects of the different levels of education on the development of critical thinking over an academic year. She compared the critical thinking abilities of first year career ladder practical nurse students with those of pre-health science baccalaureate freshmen, and the critical thinking abilities of second year career ladder AD students with those of sophomore generic BSN students. Using a pretest/posttest design, she then studied the effect of one year of academic study on the critical thinking abilities of all the groups. Critical thinking abilities were measured by administering the WGCTA at the beginning and the end of the academic year. The groups studied were drawn from schools belonging to a career ladder consortium in which one year of study at the practical nurse level could be followed by a second year of AD study, and the AD graduates were then eligible to enter the BSN programs in the consortium at the junior level. Thus, the PN/AD track was parallel to the first two years of the generic BSN track. The sample studied consisted of 55 PN and 55 AD students, representing all of the students who completed their programs, and two groups of volunteers from larger groups, one of 38 pre-health science freshmen and the other of 29 generic BSN sophomores.

The results indicated that there were no significant differences between the WGCTA scores of the PN students and the freshmen pre-health science students in either the fall or the spring. For both the fall and the spring, the sophomore BSN students had significantly higher WGCTA scores than the AD students (p < .05). The fall pretest and spring posttest scores showed non-significant increases for each group, except the BSN group, which had a non-significant decrease. In evaluating the results of her research, Kintgen-Andrews noted that the sophomore BSN students represented a population which had been screened and selected for admission to their BSN programs. Further analysis also revealed that this volunteer sample had higher average grades and class standings than the non-volunteers in their classes. When Kintgen-Andrews divided the AD students into groups according to who did well and who did poorly on the NCLEX (the former representing students who would have been likely to progress to the BSN upper division program and the latter students who would have been unlikely to do so), the fall WGCTA scores of the better AD students were much higher than the fall scores of the combined group, although still not as high as the fall scores of the BSN students. The implication is that the differences between the groups were a result of selection, rather than of the different types of programs. This is supported by the fact that there were no significant increases in WGCTA scores from the fall to the spring for any of the groups.

Relationship of Critical Thinking to Clinical Decision Making and Moral Reasoning

The following studies also examined differences in critical thinking among different types of nursing programs. In addition, they studied the relationships between critical thinking and clinical decision making, the ability to make nursing diagnoses, and moral reasoning.

Brooks and Shepherd (1990) investigated the relationship between critical thinking skills and clinical decision-making skills in nursing of senior nursing students in diploma, AD, and RN completion, and generic BSN programs. They also compared the critical thinking skills and clinical decision-making skills of the students in each type of program. Critical thinking was measured using the WGCTA, and clinical decision making in nursing by Gover's Nursing Performance Simulation Instrument (NPSI) (cited in Brooks & Shepherd, 1990). The sample studied was a convenience sample of 50 student volunteers from each type of program: generic BSN students from four different programs, AD students from two programs, and the diploma and RN students from one program each (total n = 200).

The analysis of results indicated that the WGCTA scores of students in both types of BSN programs were significantly higher than the scores of students in the diploma and AD programs (a = .05). There were no significant differences between the WGCTA scores of the two types of BSN students. The NPSI scores of the RN students were significantly higher than the scores of all the other student groups (a = .05). A weak but significant positive relationship was found between critical thinking and clinical decision making for all programs combined (r = .25). This study supported the position that baccalaureate nursing education has a greater impact on critical thinking ability than diploma or AD education. The support for the link between critical thinking ability and clinical decision making was weaker, because although there was a positive relationship between critical thinking and decision making, the correlation coefficient was low, and the only group that was significantly better at clinical decision making was the RN students, whose skills might have been more affected by practice than by education.

Pardue (1987) investigated the differences in critical thinking ability and clinical decision-making skills among graduates of AD, diploma, BSN, and MSN nursing programs. Critical thinking was measured using the WGCTA. Clinical decision making was evaluated using a tool developed by Pardue for this study. The initial sample was a stratified random sample of 360 nurses from two large health care institutions: the final sample was 121 nurses who returned the mailed research instrument. There were 24 diploma nurses, 27 AD nurses, 33 BSN nurses, and 37 MSN nurses.

The analysis revealed that there were significant differences in critical thinking abilities among the four groups of nurses (p = .001). The BSN and MSN nurses had significantly higher WGCTA scores than the diploma and AD nurses (p = .05). There were no significant differences among the four groups in clinical decision-making abilities. These results supported the position that different levels of nursing education had different effects on critical thinking abilities and that baccalaureate education improved critical thinking more than diploma or AD education. According to Pardue (1987), a limitation of the study was the instrument used for measuring clinical decision-making skills; although initial validity and reliability were established, it was a self report instrument, and may not have measured the actual skills being studied.

The results of Kintgen-Andrews (1991), Brooks and Shepherd (1990), and Pardue (1987) indicate that there are different levels of critical thinking abilities among the different levels of nursing education, but they do not explain why. Possible explanations include that the different types of programs have different effects on students' critical thinking abilities, or that students with different abilities choose or are chosen for different types of programs, or that critical thinking ability affects who can successfully complete the different types of programs. Furthermore, the lack of strong significant differences among the groups studied for clinical decision making abilities implies that improved critical thinking does not necessarily result in improved clinical decision making.

Matthews and Gaul (1979) investigated the relationship between critical thinking and the ability to derive nursing diagnoses, and compared BSN senior students with graduate students. Critical thinking was measured using WGCTA and the ability to identify nursing diagnoses was evaluated using a researcher developed case study. The sample was identified using a purposive sampling method and consisted of 22 BSN seniors and 26 graduate students. The results indicated no significant differences between the groups in WGCTA scores (p < .02). The graduate students were able to identify significantly more nursing diagnoses than the undergraduate students (p < .008). However, there was no relationship in either group between WGCTA scores and the ability to identify nursing diagnoses (rho = −.14, p < .535).

The results of Matthews and Gaul's study (1979) imply that above the BSN level, graduate education had no significant effect on critical thinking abilities. In addition, the ability to derive nursing diagnoses was not related to critical thinking as measured by the WGCTA instrument.

Ketefian (1981) studied the relationship between critical thinking, educational preparation, and moral judgment in practicing nurses, and compared the moral judgment levels of professional and technical nurses. Critical thinking was measured using the WGCTA and moral judgment using Rest's Defining Issues Test (cited in Ketefian, 1981). Educational preparation was categorized as technical (diploma or AD: n = 36) or professional (BSN or higher: n = 43). The group studied was a convenience sample of volunteer RNs drawn from three major medical centers (n = 79).

Ketefian (1981) found that critical thinking was positively related to moral judgment (r = .53, p < .001), and that professional nurses' moral judgment scores were significantly higher than the technical nurses' scores (p < .01). Multiple regression analysis revealed that critical thinking and educational level accounted for 32.9% of the variance in moral judgment. Ketefian did not examine the relationship between critical thinking and level of preparation directly. Therefore, no conclusions can be drawn from this study about the effects of different levels of nursing education on critical thinking abilities. This study does support a positive relationship between critical thinking and moral judgment.

Fleeger (1987) conducted a study investigating the effect of baccalaureate nursing education on critical thinking and moral reasoning, using a comparative design. She also investigated the relationship between aptitude and achievement and critical thinking and moral reasoning. Critical thinking was measured using the WGCTA and moral reasoning by Rest's Defining Issues Test. Aptitude and achievement were measured by SAT scores. The sample was drawn from students in the upper three years of a five year BSN program, and consisted of three groups identified using a purposive cross-sectional method: 41 Level I students tested at the beginning of their first clinical course, 23 students in the first semester of Level II, and 27 students tested during the first and last semesters of Level III.

The analysis revealed no significant differences among the three student groups in critical thinking or moral reasoning. There was a weak but positive relationship between critical thinking and moral reasoning (r = .28, p = .004), and significant relationships between critical thinking and aptitude and achievement (r = .42, p = .000), and moral reasoning and aptitude and achievement (r = .31, p = .002). Fleeger's results (1987) did not support the position that baccalaureate nursing education improved critical thinking abilities, but suggested a relationship with moral reasoning.

The correlations found between critical thinking and moral reasoning by Ketefian (1981) and Fleeger (1987) suggest a positive relationship. One possible explanation is that critical thinking is a necessary skill for moral reasoning. However, the possibility that critical thinking and moral reasoning are independently related to one or more other factors cannot be ruled out on the basis of this research.

DISCUSSION AND FUTURE DIRECTIONS
FOR NURSING EDUCATION

After a review of the published studies, several areas of concern are identified: the inadequacy of the tools used for most of the studies, the nursing populations being studied and particularly the outcome criteria that are used as variables.

Of the 13 nursing studies found in the literature, 12 used the WGCTA as at least one of the dependent variables. In the Ninth Mental Measurements Yearbook, Mitchell (1985) points out several limitations of the tool. The test measures critical thinking only through reading and does not look at the possibility that a similar score would be obtained by listening. Mitchell also feels that the test is too narrow and has a combination of neutral and controversial content that is difficult to identify. Reliability, although seen as adequate, is not as high as other cognitive tests, and construct validity is not as thorough and systematic as it could be.

Watson and Glaser (1980) report high correlations with general intelligence, yet norming data have not provided cases with an inverse relationship between intelligence and critical thinking. Since this does not occur, critical thinking as a general ability that can be measured independently of content or knowledge of the subject is questionable (McPeck, 1985).

McMillan (1987) asserts that to improve research in the area of critical thinking, rather than using the WGCTA, the tool used should closely coincide with what the intervention seeks to change. He further posits that if students begin college or a course with high scores on a measure of critical thinking, it is likely that interventions will not statistically improve the scores because the instruments currently in use may not be sufficiently difficult nor discriminating enough to measure changes.

A tool to measure critical thinking that is content specific to nursing needs to be developed. The tool needs to have a set of multiple measures of critical thinking. McMillan (1987) suggested that any tool being developed currently to measure critical thinking should take into account current philosophical definitions of critical thinking, including thinking in the context of everyday problems and decision-making situations, meta-cognitive skills, and critical thinking skills that are specific to content domain.

Another way to enhance research in the area of critical thinking would be to use more than one tool. McMillan (1987) suggested that what is needed is "greater specification of what thinking skills are being developed, with specific measurement of those skills" (p. 14). Using the tool that Ennis and Millman (1985) developed would add another possible dimension to our understanding of critical thinking. Exploring critical thinking within the framework of Perry's scheme of cognitive development using tools such as the KneWi could enhance our understanding of critical thinking. In addition the development of nursing specific tools would improve our ability to measure critical thinking in nursing.

Another problem with the populations being studied in nursing education research is that the studies have not controlled for the critical thinking abilities that students have before entering the nursing program. It is highly likely that some students have learned critical thinking skills in their previous educational and development experiences. Therefore, it is not clear what the effect of nursing education is on the development of critical thinking skills. It can be conjectured that nurses who seek higher education beyond the basic entry level are those who already have better critical thinking skills, think more independently, and/or are more intelligent. The studies that show that critical thinking increases with higher education may actually be measuring this phenomenon as opposed to the effect of the educational process.

The majority of nursing research studies on critical thinking attempt to validate the belief by the professional organizations that the difference between a technical nurse and the professional nurse is the ability to think critically. The outcome measure most commonly used to measure success in nursing education is a passing score on the NCLEX Examination. This examination is a measure of knowledge of basic nursing skills and facts, including the nursing process, but it does not directly address the area of critical thinking skills. Therefore, research in this area needs to focus on what is the goal of nursing education and how critical thinking relates to that goal.

FUTURE RESEARCH DIRECTIONS

Qualitative as well as quantitative research is needed so that nurse educators can begin to know how nursing students think both in the clinical area and in the classroom. Educators need to determine what kinds of thinking skills are necessary for nursing students to be successful in the classroom and in the clinical area and what kind of teaching strategies foster this thinking. This knowledge would allow for incorporation of these concepts into curriculum development, teaching strategies and evaluation. Miller and Malcolm (1990) suggest, for example, that by requiring students to do things in a preferred way or by making clinical errors a humiliating ordeal, educators are discouraging creativity and critical thinking.

Clear operational definitions of terms like problem solving, thinking, reasoning, clinical judgment, and critical thinking need to be developed so that research in the areas of clinical judgment, creative problem solving, and critical thinking can be organized to form a meaningful body of knowledge for the profession. This would allow for the development of a theoretical framework that could be tested and would explain why a particular experience or situation could enhance critical thinking. This would provide educators with guidance in structuring learning experiences that would enhance critical thinking.

Research Questions

Questions which need to be answered include: (1) Which curriculum best stimulates or develops critical thinking skills? (2) How should nursing incorporate the teaching of discipline specific critical thinking abilities into the curriculum? (3) Should nursing curriculum be based on critical thinking theory rather than didactic theory? (4) Does a general course in critical thinking influence critical thinking or clinical decision making in nursing? (5) Do faculty have critical thinking skills? (6) Do faculty know how to teach critical thinking? (7) What particular teaching method or style influences critical thinking in nursing students? (8) Does the Socratic method of instruction enhance critical thinking skills in nursing students? (9) What kind of clinical activities should be designed for students to enhance critical thinking skills? (10) Does conducting research or learning the research process teach or stimulate critical thinking? (11) Are technical and professional students different? (12) Is technical and professional education different?

CONCLUSION

The pace of change in the area of health care is accelerating at a remarkable rate. It is the responsibility of nurse educators to ensure that nursing graduates have developed the critical thinking abilities necessary to practice the profession of nursing. We need to abandon educational methods that make students passive recipients of information and adopt those that transform them into active participants in their own intellectual growth. "When we teach each subject in such a way that students pass courses without thinking their way into the knowledge that these subjects make possible, students leave those courses without any more knowledge than when they entered them. When we sacrifice thought to gain coverage, we sacrifice knowledge at the same time. The issue is not shall we sacrifice knowledge to spend time on thought, but shall we continue to sacrifice both knowledge and thought for the mere appearance of learning" (Paul, 1990, p. 47).

Research into the way nurses process information has started building a body of knowledge that is specific to the profession of nursing (Broderick & Ammentorp, 1979; Matthews & Gaul, 1979; Westfall, Tanner, Putzier, & Padrick, 1986). Future research in the area of critical thinking should focus on proving that nurses not only know what to think, but also know how to think.

REFERENCES

Anderson, J. (1961). Socrates as an educator. In J. Anderson (Ed.), *Studies in imperial philosophy.* Sidney, Australia: Angus & Robertson.

Aristotle. (1962). *Nicomachean ethics.* (M. Oswald, Trans.) New York: Bobbs-Merrill.

Aune, B. (1967). *Thinking: Encyclopedia of philosophy.* (Vol. 8, pp. 100–104). New York: Macmillan.

Bauwens, E., & Gerhard, G. (1987). The use of the Watson-Glaser Critical Thinking Appraisal to predict success in a baccalaureate nursing program. *Journal of Nursing Education 26,* 278–281.

Berger, M. (1984). Clinical thinking ability and nursing students. *Journal of Nursing Education, 23,* 306–308.

Broderick, M. E., & Ammentorp, W. (1979). Information structures: An analysis of nursing performance. *Nursing Research, 28,* 106–110.

Brooks, K. L., & Shepherd, J. M. (1990). The relationship between clinical decision-making skills in nursing and general critical thinking abilities of senior nursing students in four types of nursing programs. *Journal of Nursing Education, 2,* 391–399.

Dewey, J. (1916). *Democracy and education: An introduction to the philosophy of education.* New York: Macmillan.

Ennis, R. (1985). A logical basis for measuring critical thinking skills. *Educational Leadership, 43,* 44–48.

Ennis, R. (1989). Critical thinking and subject specificity: Clarification and needed research. *Educational Researcher, 18*(3), 4–10.

Ennis, Robert H., & Millman, J. (1985). *Cornell tests of critical thinking.* Pacific Grove, CA: Midwest.

Facione, P. (1984). Toward a theory of critical thinking. *Liberal Education, 70,* 253–256.

Fleeger, R. L. (1987). Critical thinking and moral reasoning behavior of baccalaureate nursing students (Abstract). *Proceedings of the Fifth Annual Research in Nursing Education Conference, 5,* 34.

Furedy, C., & Furedy, J. (1985). Critical thinking: Toward research and dialogue. In J. G. Donald & A. M. Sullivan (Eds.), *Using research to improve thinking: New directions for teaching and learning.* San Francisco: Jossey-Bass.

Glaser, E. (1941). *An experiment in the development of critical thinking.* New York: Teachers College of Columbia University.

Gross, Y., Takazawa, E., & Rose, C. (1987). Critical thinking and nursing education. *Journal of Nursing Education, 26,* 317–323.

Halpern, D. (1984). *Thought and knowledge.* Hillsdale, NJ: Lawrence Erlbaum.

Ketefian, S. (1981). Critical thinking, educational preparation, and development of moral judgment among selected groups of practicing nurses. *Nursing Research, 30,* 98–103.

Kintgen-Andrews, J. (1988). Development of critical thinking: Career ladder PN and AD nursing students, pre-health science freshmen, generic baccalaureate sophomore nursing students. *Resources in Education, 24*(1). (ERIC Document No. ED 297 153).

Kintgen-Andrews, J. (1991). Critical thinking and nursing education: Perplexities and insights. *Journal of Nursing Education, 30,* 152–157.

Kurfiss, J. G. (1988). *Critical thinking: Theory, research, practice, and possibilities.* (ASHE-ERIC Higher Education Report No. 2.) Washington, DC: Association for Study of Higher Education.

Lynch, M. (1988). Critical thinking: A comparative study of baccalaureate and associate degree nursing students. (Doctoral dissertation, George Peabody College for Teachers) *Dissertation Abstracts International, 49,* 2157A.

Matthews, C., & Gaul, A. (1979). Nursing diagnosis from the perspective of concept attainment and critical thinking. *Advances in Nursing Science, 2,* 17–26.

McMillan, J. (1987). Enhancing college students' critical thinking: A review of studies. *Research in Higher Education, 26*(1), 3–29.

McPeck, J. E. (1985). Critical thinking and the "Trivial Pursuit" theory of knowledge. *Teaching Philosophy, 8,* 295–308.

Miller, M., & Malcolm, N. S. (1990). Critical thinking in the nursing curriculum. *Nursing and Health Care, 11,* 66–73.

Mitchell, J. (1985). *The ninth mental measurements yearbook.* Lincoln, NE: The Burrows Institute of Mental Measurements.

Norris, S. (1985). Synthesis of research on critical thinking. *Educational Leadership, 2*(8), 40–45.

Pardue, S. F. (1987). Decision-making skills and critical thinking ability among associate degree, diploma, baccalaureate, and master's prepared nurses. *Journal of Nursing Education 26,* 354–361.

Paul, R. (1990). *Critical thinking. What every person needs to know to survive in a rapidly changing world.* Rohnert Park, CA: Sonoma State University.

Perry, W. G. (1970). *Forms of intellectual and ethical development in the college years:* A scheme. New York: Holt, Rinehart.

Sullivan, E. (1987). Critical thinking, creativity, clinical performance, and achievements in RN students. *Nurse Educator, 12*(2), 12–16.

Tiessen, J. B. (1987). Critical thinking and selected correlates among baccalaureate nursing students. *Journal of Professional Nursing, 3,* 118–123.

Valiga, T. M. (1983). Cognitive development: A critical component of baccalaureate nursing education. *Image, 15*(4), 115–119.

Watson, G., & Glaser, E. (1964). *Critical thinking appraisal manual.* New York: Harcourt. Brace & World.

Watson, G., & Glaser, E. (1980). *Critical thinking manual.* Dallas, TX: Psychological Corporation.

Westfall, U., Tanner, C., Putzier, D. and Padrick, K. (1986). Activating clinical inferences: A component of diagnostic reasoning in nursing. *Research in Nursing and Health, 9,* 269–277.

Widick, C. A. (1975). The Perry scheme: A foundation for developmental practice. *The Counseling Psychologist, 6,* 35–38.

Chapter Two

NONTRADITIONAL STUDENTS IN HIGHER EDUCATION: A REVIEW OF THE LITERATURE AND IMPLICATIONS FOR NURSING EDUCATION

Cesarina M. Thompson, MS, RN

INTRODUCTION

Much has been written about the use of the andragogical approach in teaching adult learners (Apps, 1981; Brookfield, 1986; Knowles, 1980). These adult learning concepts have been described frequently in the nursing literature, particularly in relation to teaching RN-BSN students (Baj, 1985; Dyck, 1986; Fotos, 1987). However, there is a lack of empirical evidence supporting the use of andragogical principles with adult nursing students (basic non-nurse students and RNs) in higher education. Although the andragogical approach may indeed be effective with adults in continuing education or other non-degree programs, alternative frameworks for working with adult nursing students in colleges and universities need to be considered. In this chapter, then, I will describe the andragogical approach, review literature related to the use of andragogy with adults in general and adult nursing students in particular, discuss the implications of the literature for nursing education, and pose additional questions for nursing research.

PRINCIPLES OF ANDRAGOGY

Adult educators agree that the learning needs of adults are quite different than those of younger students (Knowles, 1980; Knox, 1986). These needs are generally reflective of the developmental differences between traditional and nontraditional or adult students. Traditional students are usually full-time students

31

between 18 and 24 years of age. Nontraditional students are usually over the age of 24, enroll in institutions of higher education as part-time students, and fulfill several life roles in addition to their roles as students (e.g., parent, worker).

In addition, adults usually enter colleges and universities with a wealth of life and work experiences from which they have derived specific goals and objectives. The literature indicates that adults return to school primarily to improve their current job skills or to acquire new skills (Cross, 1981). In contrast, traditional students usually enter institutions of higher education with limited life and work experiences and look to the institution to provide them with the knowledge they will eventually need as productive citizens.

Due to these basic differences, adult educators support the use of the andragogical approach with adult learners. According to Knowles (1980), andragogy can be defined as the "art and science of helping adults learn" (p. 43). Specific assumptions underlying andragogy include recognizing the experiences of adults as a rich resource for learning, adults as self-directed learners, and adults as having problem-oriented learning needs.

Using andragogy as a framework, educators of adults should create a supportive learning environment, use learners' experience as a resource for learning, encourage students to collaborate and participate in the learning process (Brookfield, 1986). The successful educator of adults should ground learning activities in the learners' experiences and help students make connections between the new knowledge introduced and their own experiences. In addition, adult educators should encourage students to be self-directed, respond to learners' needs, and respect diverse ways of learning (Apps, 1981; Knox, 1986). Teaching strategies, such as discussion and role playing, are seen as superior to the traditional lecture method because they call upon the learners' experience and encourage students to participate actively in the learning process.

REVIEW OF LITERATURE

Although much can be found in the literature supporting the use of the andragogical approach with adult learners, few have studied the effect of using these principles on learning outcomes of adult students. While adults differ from traditional students in relation to age and in the number of roles they fulfill, are they really different as learners?

Beder and Carrea (1988) conducted a randomized control group field experiment using treatment, placebo, and null groups to identify if teachers of adults trained in the use of andragogical techniques would have higher rates of student attendance in their classes and if their students would report a higher rate of satisfaction. The hypothesis that students of teachers who had received training in adult learning techniques would be more satisfied and have a higher rate of attendance than students of teachers who did not receive such training was not supported. Another study focusing on adults in a continuing education program explored the effect of adult learner participation in planning the program on student achievement and satisfaction (Rosenblum & Darkenwald, 1983). Findings showed that participation did not result in higher achievement and satisfaction. Interestingly, those who did not participate (control group) scored higher on both achievement and satisfaction.

Adults in Higher Education

The number of adult learners in institutions of higher education is steadily increasing. It is estimated that by 1992 adult learners over the age of 25 will comprise half of the student population on college and university campuses (Lynton & Elman, 1987). Despite the growing number of adult students in institutions of higher education, there is a dearth of research focusing on effective teaching strategies for adult learners. However, the available literature suggests that the principles of andragogy may not be effective for adults in colleges and universities. In fact, only one study's findings supported the use of andragogical techniques.

Conti and Welborn (1986) studied the effect of the collaborative approach on the achievement scores of adults enrolled in college courses. The authors concluded that the teaching style significantly affected learning, and that the use of the collaborative mode resulted in the greatest student achievement.

In contrast, Tracy and Schuttenberg (1986) found that the majority of adult learners enrolled in college courses perceived the instructor to be the expert and to know more than the learner in terms of course planning. In addition, while some adult learners favored collaboration in course planning, they indicated that their preference for this mode would depend on the type of course being offered. This study indicates that not all adults prefer teaching strategies reflective of andragogical principles. The authors suggest that there are several factors which may influence teaching preferences, such as past experiences, locus of control, and self-concept as a learner.

Similarly, Loesch and Foley (1988) surveyed 63 adult learners enrolled in traditional and non-traditional baccalaureate programs, giving each the Learning Preference Inventory (LPI). Findings showed that while some adults preferred student-structured learning reflective of self-directedness, others preferred teacher-structured learning.

Werring (1984) compared 731 traditional college students and 563 non-traditional students for their teaching preferences. Results showed that there were no significant differences between traditional and non-traditional students in their preference for structured learning and independent learning situations. These findings do not support the widely accepted assumption that adults are self-directed learners. Interestingly, differences in instructional preferences were found to be related not to the age of the students, but to their status in the undergraduate program. Specifically, upper division students were more likely to prefer independent study modes than lower division students.

Ross (1989) surveyed 181 undergraduate adult students enrolled in one university to identify their perception of best and worst instructional practices. Clarity of presentation, eliciting student participation, and interesting and organized lectures were frequently reported as best instructional practices. These findings do not support existing literature on adult learners which discourages the use of the lecture format and teacher dominance in the classroom.

Adult Learners in Nursing

Although much can be found in the nursing literature supporting the use of andragogical techniques with adult learners, empirical evidence is lacking. The majority of articles supporting the use of these principles focus on RNs in continuing education programs (Smith, 1978; Tibbles, 1977; Wolanin, 1979). However, results from a recent study conducted by Russell (1990) are not consistent with the existing literature in this area.

Russell (1990) explored the relationship among educational structure (high or low structure), self-directed learning readiness

(SDLR), instructional methods (lecture or module), and achievement. The sample consisted of 40 RNs involved in a hospital based continuing education program on arterial blood gases. Participants were tested for their educational structure preference and SDLR. Following testing, subjects were randomly assigned to either the lecture or module method. Results showed that no relationship existed between the variables being studied. Specifically, the posttest performance of subjects who preferred high structure was not affected by the type of instructional method (lecture or module) they received. The same was found to be true for subjects who preferred low structure.

In relation to higher education, most of the literature focuses on teaching RNs in BSN programs (Baj, 1985; Beeman, 1988; Dyck, 1986). Only two studies could be found that explored the teaching preferences of nontraditional students in baccalaureate nursing programs. Seidl and Sauter (1990) found that although traditional and non-traditional nursing students differed in terms of learning style, no difference existed regarding students' preferred teaching methods.

Similarly, Linares (1989) found no significant difference between traditional nursing students and RNs in a baccalaureate program in relation to their self-directed learning readiness.

While definitive conclusions cannot be drawn from a limited number of studies, the existing evidence from educational and nursing research suggests that nontraditional students are not significantly different than generic or traditional students with respect to their preferences for teaching methods.

A study by Bueche (1986) comparing the developmental patterns of re-entry women (non-RNs) and generic students in baccalaureate nursing programs may partially explain why the use of adult learning techniques for nontraditional nursing students does not necessarily result in higher achievement and/or satisfaction. Using the Developmental Task Inventory, Bueche surveyed 156 traditional age and 50 re-entry women in baccalaureate nursing programs in six public institutions. Results showed that while re-entry students scored significantly higher than generic students on Task I (Developing Autonomy), no significant differences were found between the two groups in relation to Task II (Developing Purpose) and Task III (Developing Mature Interpersonal Relationships). Hence, findings from this study do not support the existing literature which suggests that adults are developmentally different learners than traditional students and thus, should be taught differently.

In a similar vein, King (1986) compared the developmental patterns of RNs and generic students in a baccalaureate nursing program. Students were compared in terms of three factors: life stage, ego development, and learning style. Although no significant differences were found between RNs and generic students in relation to learning style, significant differences were found in life stage and ego development. While generic students were in the developmental stage of Early Adult Transition, RNs were dealing with the Age 30 Transition or the Mid-life Transition (King, 1986). The author concluded that RN students in the study were substantially different than generic students in relation to adult development.

Although RNs in the study by King (1986) were found to be at different life stages than generic students in terms of career development, and family and work responsibilities, are the two groups significantly different as learners? Existing evidence, although limited, does not seem to support the concept that traditional and nontraditional students differ significantly with respect to their preferences for teaching methods. In addition, the instructional methods used do not seem to affect learning outcomes for adult students. Studies focusing on nontraditional students in higher education are summarized in Table 1. Studies focusing on nontraditional nursing students (basic non-nurses and RNs) are summarized in Table 2.

IMPLICATIONS FOR NURSING EDUCATION

Re-entry into higher education can be a stressful period for adults. The literature indicates that many adults enter colleges and universities with much concern about their ability to succeed (Cross, 1981). This concern with ability may be related to several factors, such as poor past experiences with educational settings, poorly developed sense of self, and lack of social support for educational pursuits (Cross, 1981).

In addition, adults facing this transitional period in their development may find themselves questioning their choices in life and revising their goals and objectives. According to life events and transitions theorists (e.g., Lowenthal, Thurnher, & Chiriboga), the event or transition an individual is facing is more important than his or her age. Life events theorists believe that the issues related to a particular event in life are the same for all individuals

Table 2. Research Studies on Adult Students in Nursing Programs

Study	Description	Variables	Findings
Bueche, 1986	Compared developmental patterns of nontrad. (non-RNs) & generic nursing students	Developmental stage	Significant differences found only on Task I (Autonomy). No differences found in 2 other tasks: Developing Purpose & Developing Mature Interpersonal Relationships
King, 1986	Developmental patterns of RNs & generic nursing students	Developmental stage	Generic students were in Early Adult Transition & RNs were in Age 30 Transition
Linares, 1989	Compared RNs & traditional students for self-directed learning readiness (SDLR)	SDLR level	No significant difference between groups
Merritt, 1983	Learning style of traditional & non-traditional students	Learning style	Style of non-traditional students not reflective of adult learning theory
Russell, 1990	Studied effect of 2 teaching methods on achievement of RNs	Educational structure, SDLR, teaching method, achievement	Achievement not affected by teaching method
Seidl & Sauter, 1990	Explored preferred teaching methods of traditional & non-traditional nursing students	Preferred teaching method	No significant difference found between groups

Table 1. Research Studies on Adults in Higher Education

Study	Description	Variables	Findings
Conti & Welborn, 1986	Studied effect of teaching method on achievement of adults in college courses	Collaborative teaching method, Achievement	Collaborative mode yielded higher achievement
Loesch & Foley, 1988	Teaching preferences of 63 adult college students	Teaching preference	Not all students preferred self-directedness
Ross, 1989	Surveyed 181 adult college students for best & worst teaching practices	Teaching practices	Preferences reflective of traditional methods
Tracy & Schuttenberg, 1986	Survey of adult college students' preferences	Teaching preferences	Majority preferred teacher structured setting
Werring, 1984	Compared 731 traditional college students and 563 adult students for teaching preferences	Teaching preferences	Preferences related to stage in educational program, not age of student

experiencing that event regardless of their age (Schlossberg, 1984). Hence, adults in institutions of higher education may be facing the same issues (e.g., purpose in life, career goals, etc.) as generic students. Although chronologically adult learners in nursing (RNs and non-nurses) may be older than generic students, as learners, some may be in the earlier stages of development. Thus, nursing educators cannot assume that the andragogical approach should be used with all adult learners because of their age and stage in life. An alternative approach to teaching adults is to consider each learner individually with respect to factors, such as self-concept as a learner, life transitions, and past experiences (Cross, 1981).

A supportive learning environment which provides adult students with guidance and direction, at least in the initial stages of their educational experience, may be a much more effective strategy than promoting self-direction. As students progress through the educational program, strategies which require more independence could then be introduced. As shown in the study by Werring (1984), regardless of their age, upper division students were more likely to prefer independent learning activities than lower division students. Thus, planning teaching strategies according to the students' stage in the educational program may result in higher academic achievement.

Another factor to consider when working with adult learners is the concept of learning styles. The literature reviewed indicates that differences in learning preferences can be identified in both traditional and nontraditional students. Not all adult learners prefer instructional methods that promote self-directedness. Even (1982) notes that the andragogical approach advocates the use of strategies that are appropriate only for learners who prefer self-directed learning. Merritt (1983) surveyed 343 basic and RN students enrolled in six generic BSN programs for learning style preferences using Kolb's and Canfield's learning style models. Findings showed that while some differences in learning style preference did exist between traditional and nontraditional students, these differences were not reflective of adult learning theory. Interestingly, both groups, traditional and nontraditional, preferred structured learning environments. In addition, neither group showed a preference for self-directedness (i.e., setting own learning goals) in the learning environment. Results of this study further support that the age of the learner should not be the primary factor in determining choice of teaching methods.

Kolb's Experiential Learning Model (Kolb, 1984) may be a more effective approach to teaching adult learners. While this model acknowledges the learner's experience as a basis for learning, it also forces the learner to process information using four distinct modes. The four modes identified in the model are: concrete experience, reflective observation, abstract conceptualization, and active experimentation. Kolb's Learning Style Inventory (LSI) can be used to identify the dominant learning mode for each individual. However, Kolb maintains that for learners to be successful they must be able to process information in all four modes. Hence, instructional methods for adult learners should not be limited by the andragogical principles which advocate basing instruction on the learning needs and experiences of the learner. Educators of adults should help students analyze and challenge new ideas vis a vis their existing knowledge.

Finally, the concept of motivation to learn has not been addressed in the studies reviewed. Literature in the area of motivation suggests that motivation does affect learning. A motivated learner will usually perform at a higher level than the unmotivated learner (Wlodkowski, 1988). Hence, the instructional method used may have little, if any, effect on achievement if the learner does not want to learn. Six major factors of motivation have been identified: attitude, need, stimulation, affect, competence, and reinforcement. Successful educators of adults should plan instructional strategies which address all of these factors in order to enhance motivation to learn. Wlodkowski's Time Continuum Model describes three critical periods in any learning sequence: Beginning, during, and ending. Motivational strategies specific to each phase of the learning cycle are identified in the model. Educators can use this model to maximize the motivation of learners and ultimately affect achievement.

RECOMMENDATIONS FOR NURSING RESEARCH

Review of educational and nursing literature indicates that the use of andragogical teaching methods with nontraditional students is a widely accepted practice. However, empirical evidence supporting this practice with nontraditional students in higher education is lacking. Considering the increasing number of nontraditional students (adult non-nurses and RNs) in baccalaureate nursing programs, future studies in nursing education should address the following questions:

1. Which teaching methods are effective with nontraditional students in baccalaureate nursing programs?
2. Does the use of andragogical techniques result in higher adult student achievement when compared with the use of traditional teaching methods?

In addition, to expand our knowledge base of the teaching-learning process, studies focusing on other variables identified in the literature to affect adult learning should also be conducted. One important factor noted to influence adult learning is motivation. It would be interesting to explore if a high level of motivation results in higher academic achievement regardless of the teaching methods used.

REFERENCES

Apps, J. W. (1981). *The adult learner on campus.* Chicago: Follett Publishing.

Baj, P. (1985). Can the generic curriculum function for the returning RN student? *Journal of Nursing Education, 24,* 69–71.

Beder, H., & Carrea, N. (1988). The effects of andragogical teacher training on adult students' attendance and evaluation of their teachers. *Adult Education Quarterly, 38,* 75–87.

Beeman, P. (1988). RNs' perceptions of their baccalaureate programs: Meeting their adult learning needs. *Journal of Nursing Education, 27,* 364–370.

Brookfield, S. (1986). *Understanding and facilitating adult learning.* San Francisco: Jossey-Bass.

Bueche, M. N. (1986). Re-entry women in baccalaureate nursing programs: The achievement of selected developmental tasks. *Journal of Nursing Education, 25,* 15–19.

Conti, G., & Welborn, R. (1986). Teaching-learning styles and the adult learner. *Life-Long Learning, 9,* 20–24.

Cross, K. P. (1981). *Adults as learners.* San Francisco: Jossey-Bass.

Dyck, S. (1986). Self-directed learning for the RN in a baccalaureate program. *Journal of Continuing Education in Nursing, 17,* 194–197.

Even, M. J. (1982). Adapting cognitive style theory in practice. *Life-Long Learning, 5,* 14–17, 27.

Fotos, J. (1987). Characteristics of RN students continuing their education in a B.S. program. *Journal of Continuing Education in Nursing, 18,* 118–122.

King, J. E. (1986). A comparative study of adult developmental patterns of RN and generic students in a baccalaureate nursing program. *Journal of Nursing Education, 25,* 366–371.

Knowles, M. S. (1980). *The modern practice of adult education: From pedagogy to andragogy.* New York: Cambridge.

Knox, A. B. (1986). *Helping adults learn.* San Francisco: Jossey-Bass.

Kolb, D. A. (1984). *Experiential learning: Experience as the source of learning and development.* Englewood Cliffs: Prentice-Hall.

Linares, A. Z. (1989). A comparative study of learning characteristics of RN and generic students. *Journal of Nursing Education, 28,* 354–359.

Loesch, T., & Foley, R. (1988). Learning preference differences among adults in traditional and nontraditional baccalaureate programs. *Adult Education Quarterly, 38,* 224–233.

Lynton, E. A., & Elman, S. E. (1987). *New priorities for the university.* San Francisco: Jossey-Bass.

Merritt, S. L. (1983). Learning style preferences of baccalaureate nursing students. *Nursing Research, 32,* 367–372.

Rosenblum, S., & Darkenwald, G. (1983). Effects of adult learners participation in course planning on achievement and satisfaction. *Adult Education Quarterly, 33,* 147–153.

Ross, J. M. (1989, March). *Critical teaching behaviors as perceived by adult undergraduates.* Paper presented at the Annual Meeting of the American Educational Research Association, San Francisco, CA.

Russell, J. M. (1990). Relationships among preference for educational structure, self-directed learning, instructional methods, and achievement. *Journal of Professional Nursing, 6,* 86–93.

Schlossberg, N. K. (1984). *Counseling adults in transition.* New York: Springer.

Seidl, A. H., & Sauter, D. (1990). The new non-traditional student in nursing. *Journal of Nursing Education, 29,* 13–19.

Smith, C. (1978). Principles and implications for continuing education in nursing. *Journal of Continuing Education in Nursing, 9*(2), 25–28.

Tibbles, L. (1977). Theories of adult education: Implications for continuing education in nursing. *Journal of Continuing Education in Nursing, 8*(4), 25–28.

Tracy, S., & Schuttenberg, E. (1986). Exploring adult learners' rationale for course interaction preferences. *Adult Education Quarterly, 36,* 142–156.

Werring, C. (1984). *A comparison of preferences toward the curriculum and instruction process of traditional and older aged undergraduate students at Texas Technical University* (Doctoral Dissertation, University of Georgia, 1984). Pub. No. AAC8427590.

Wlodkowski, R. J. (1988). *Enhancing adult motivation to learn.* San Francisco: Jossey-Bass.

Wolanin, M. (1973). Factors leading to effectiveness of continuing education programs. *Journal of Continuing Education in Nursing, 4*(6), 14–19.

Chapter Three

QUALITATIVE RESEARCH IN NURSING EDUCATION

Helen J. Streubert, EdD, RN
Joan M. Jenks, PhD, RN

INTRODUCTION

This review describes how nurse educators to date have incorporated qualitative research in their quest for knowledge. Since the term *qualitative research* can be vague and ambiguous, here it is defined as a collection of research methodologies that share several basic beliefs: theory building is inductive; control of researcher bias is impossible and unnecessary; and both context and subjectivity are essential to the understanding of phenomenon under study. Of the qualitative research methodologies included in this review, all specify this objective: the description of aspects of nursing education completed for understanding, not prediction of human behavior.

The 45 qualitative research studies reviewed here represent at least five distinct qualitative methodologies: phenomenology (used most), naturalistic inquiry, case study, grounded theory, and ethnography. The researchers who reported using phenomenology have indicated a variety of approaches which are highlighted in the reporting of the study if they were identified by the author(s). Five studies only report the use of qualitative methods without an identification of any specific methodology. Each study's method will be described as the researcher has identified it. The 20 unpublished studies reviewed here were conducted as doctoral dissertations. As such, their review is based on their published abstract, limiting our methodological critique.

The studies reviewed will be categorized by informants involved: students; faculty; academic administrators; curriculum planners; and staff development educators. The review begins with a discussion of the contribution of qualitative studies involving nursing students.

STUDENTS

Students' Lived Experiences

A category of studies emerges whose primary focus has been the study of students' lived experiences. These studies have not been directed at one particular aspect of the students' experience, such as their perceptions of being cared for, but rather, have been directed at understanding the students' experiences of their education. Six studies have been completed that provide insight into the experience of nursing students.

Nelms (1990) conducted a phenomenological study of 17 nursing students at Georgia State University. Interview questions were developed by the researcher to guide data collection. Nelms identified categories common to each student's experience: life-pervasive commitment; the meaning of clinical; personal knowledge experiences; support systems; feelings about myself; and ideal teacher.

The theme life-pervasive commitment in this study reflects students' knowledge of the level of commitment they have accepted by their entry into professional nursing. The amount of information they must master is perceived to be time consuming and requires them to attend to it with intensity. Their clinical experience is seen as the "single most meaningful aspect of their lived experiences" (Nelms, 1990, p. 289). The meaning of *clinical* is important as it gives value to their lives as students. Informants shared how their personal knowledge informed their lives as students, and how their support systems (fellow classmates, faculty, and staff nurses) as well as their feelings about themselves and their perceptions of ideal teacher shaped their respective experiences.

Interested in knowing what nursing students think about nursing, Melia (1982) conducted a study using grounded theory. Forty informal interviews were completed and then transcribed. Categories common to these students' experiences included: learning and working; getting the work done; learning the rules; nursing in the dark; just passing through; and doing nursing and being professional. In the article reviewed, Melia offers only part of the complete study, focusing on what "nursing in the dark" is for the students in her study. As a category of data, nursing in the dark reflects students' concerns about what they could and could not say to patients. Her informants felt ill informed about specific patient care information and at times about the patient's diagnosis. This lead Melia to conclude that her informants frequently perceived that they were "nursing in the dark." Melia states: "Whilst this study arrives at no theory which can be stated in a concise way, the conceptual categories are offered as a means of describing and explaining the student nurses' accounts of their work and training (p. 334)."

Bush (1976) provides a description of male nursing students' experiences. Her study purported: "to investigate how and why men decide to become nurses; which forces in society are inhibiting, which are encouraging; and how these forces are perceived and accommodated in the effort to maximize social benefits and minimize social costs (p. 393)."

Focused interviews were conducted with ten male nurses. Eight of these were students: four undergraduate and four graduate. Of the remaining two, one was a faculty member and the other was employed full-time in a university hospital. An interview guide with 17 probe questions was used to trigger the memory of the informants and give structure to the conversation. Specifically, questions addressed the past, present, and future, including: "Why do you think men enter nursing? Do you think most male nurses felt they were going to be stigmatized? Do you feel you are treated differently by others? Do you think male nurses stick together? Do you think your career expectations are limited, enhanced or different because you are a male?" (Bush, 1984, pp. 404–405).

Findings were reported purely as descriptions of the informants' dialogue with the researcher. No theme categories were identified. The researcher suggested, "in the absence of cultural definition of their status, male aspirants to nursing must develop coping skills that facilitate acceptable definitions of themselves" (Bush, 1976, p. 402). Further, "role strain can be reduced by the selection of specialities that do not require giving personal care and in which non-traditional clothing may be worn" (p. 403).

Van Dongen (1988) provides insight into the live experiences of full-time doctoral students. The data collection methods included participant observation, in-depth semi-structured interviews, and two 24-hour logs of the investigator's experience as a student and researcher. Student participants included seven first-year students, including the researcher. Data were analyzed using comparative analysis. "The conceptual categories which emerged were: impact, changes, losses, uncertainty, stressors, vulnerability, stress response, coping mechanisms, situation supports, commitment,

and outcomes" (p. 21). The categories reflect the students' perceptions of what the experience of being a doctoral student is: the
impact of the experience; how they are required to make changes
in their lives; the losses they must accept such as loss of earning
power while a student; the uncertainty that comes with returning
to school and seeing themselves in new roles; the stressors and how
they cope; and their enduring commitment to achieve their desired
personal outcomes.

Van Dongen (1988) concludes her study by stating that findings
provide a "detailed description of the human experience of beginning full-time doctoral study" (p. 24). As she recommends, additional studies in other university environments will further the
understanding of doctoral students' experiences. Although the
data reported are limited, the study does provide prospective doctoral students and graduate level educators with insight into how
it is to live the doctoral student experience.

Kayser-Jones and Abu-Saad (1982) provide an example of a
study using qualitative data to develop a measure to determine the
difficulties foreign students encounter upon entering a strange
culture to obtain their education. These researchers were interested in identifying "the difficulties international nursing students
experience in adjusting to American culture and to university
nursing programs, and to elucidate those factors that would facilitate students' adjustments" (pp. 304–305). "Open-ended, qualitative responses" (p. 305) were sought during interviews conducted
with 26 foreign nursing students with the specific intent of con-
structing major categories toward development of an instrument.
From the data collected, a questionnaire consisting of 43 fixed
alternative and open-ended questions in the major categories of
student difficulties in adjustment to the nursing program and university, factors which enhanced adjustment to American culture,
factors effecting classroom learning and factors effecting clinical
learning was developed. The overriding theme throughout the
students' descriptions of their experiences was loneliness. Based
on their findings, the researchers suggest several recommenda-
tions to enhance the experience of foreign nursing students. These
include developing "international companion programs" (p. 311)
that would assist foreign students in establishing friendships, and
developing international nursing organizations with the purpose
of bringing together foreign students and American faculty to
discuss national and international nursing issues. Other recom-
mendations include developing a course that would promote

"understanding of cultural beliefs, customs and values" (p. 312) and establishing host families with whom foreign students could live.

Field (1981) was interested in a phenomenological view of one aspect of clinical experience: the experience of giving an injection. To that end, she interviewed nursing students, nurses, and patients. Her specific focus involved the individuals who had administered injections. Ten of the informants were undergraduate nursing students, ten experienced nurses, and four were diabetic patients. Participants' experiences were collected by essays and interviews. Field reported her findings in four major categories, including: injections, with subcategories of the language of injections, the giver, and hurting the other; preparing for the injection; the act; response to the act; and the unconscious patient, the silent body.

The data were reported primarily in the informants' words. Field (1981) states, "the phenomenologist never reaches a conclusion . . . the essay should challenge the reader to respond by saying, 'Yes, it is like this', or 'No, I don't believe it is like that'" (p. 29). In closing, Field found that such a study may:

> . . . help educators to better understand the meaning of the anxiety that is observed as a student undertakes the act of giving her first injection, so she may help the student reflect and come to understand the meaning of that experience (p. 295).

Students' Attitudes

Grassi-Russo and Morris (1981) offer additional insight into the attitudes of nursing students. They asked 102 members of the freshmen class of a diploma school to record in one phrase or less anticipatory fears and hopes about their upcoming educational experience. Eight months after the original data collection period, students were "asked to write down the two experiences in school which were most pleasant and/or positive and the two which were most unpleasant or negative" (p. 11). Only 83 of the original participants were still in the program at the time of the second data collection.

Analysis of the data included sorting the students' responses into categories reflecting their most common fears, positive, and negative experiences. The students' responses were tabulated using rank, frequency, and percentages. From these statistical data,

the researchers identified common themes, including: compe-
tency, pressure and stress, instructor as role model, fear of failure,
and expectation of success.

Students expressed overwhelmingly their desire to feel competent, with the theme of competence implicit in their descriptions of fear of making mistakes, fear of failure, and uneasiness
with the assumption of responsibilities related to patient care. Associated with their need to feel competent was the theme of pressure and stress described as directly related to students' expected
perceptions of themselves as competent caregivers as well as with
personal needs to feel successful in their academic pursuits.

Fear of failure and expectation of success also are related to the
overall expectations for performance. Students fear low achievement and are in constant need of reinforcement that they can be
successful in their academic goals. Faculty are the individuals to
whom students look for this support. Students additionally look to
faculty as role models—another major theme. Students derive
much of their perceptions of success from seeing themselves as
professionally competent as their teachers. According to Grassi-
Russo and Morris (1981), faculty are seen not only as "exemplars
of 'grace under pressure' but also as empathic helping persons to
whom students themselves can go for support" (p. 15).

The researchers conclude that if additional studies are conducted to identify and examine freshmen students' attitudes,
"more qualified people [would] complete nursing school . . .
[and] the experience would be characterized much more by
hopes than by fears" (p. 16). Unfortunately, this conclusion is a
grand leap from the findings presented and does not seem appropriate in light of the data available to the reader.

Student Program Preference

Simms (1981) conducted a study of student preference for program type using the grounded theory approach as described by
Glaser and Strauss (1967). Research was directed toward the development of a theory about the factors that influence nurses'
preference for external degree or off-campus study in a graduate
administration program.

A sample of 23 respondents resulted from inclusion of 13 enrolled on-campus students and 10 nurses with baccalaureate preparation who sent letters of inquiry to the graduate program office in
one university. Data were collected via telephone interviews. An

interview schedule was developed to ascertain the students' educational interests. From analysis of the interviews, six categories were identified with 67 related properties. The second phase of the study included the development of a questionnaire based on the initial findings. This questionnaire was subsequently mailed to 846 nurses in Michigan. "Using the concepts, related properties, survey data analysis, and testing of the propositions, a work-study theory of preference for off-campus study was developed" (Simms, 1981, p. 359). Simms concludes that the grounded theory approach is a useful way to study nursing problems.

Role Socialization

In an admirable attempt to describe the professional socialization of nursing students in a college of nursing, Olsen and Whittaker (1968) completed an ethnographic study of one class of students during the three years of their nursing studies. The researchers used participant observation and interview to study the students in the school environment interacting with their faculty. The crucial influence of the students', the schools', and the profession's history on each student's socialization also was included. Data were analyzed from a framework of symbolic interaction. Themes describing socialization of the student include: the crucial influence of the academic setting and the faculty; students' adaptation to the role of student, especially "psyching out" the faculty; confirmation of self through interaction with fellow students, faculty, nursing staff, physicians, family, and friends; and the student's individual interpretation of the events of his or her own socialization. Use of an exhaustive methodology and detailed reporting that fully informs the reader of the student experience strengthens the study. As such, the reader has a full appreciation of socialization of this group of students. Study results are presented in sufficient detail to facilitate the reader's transference of the insights presented.

Massumi (1989) completed a dissertation which provides insight into role socialization of nursing students. Twenty-two female respondents participated in the study: 15 nursing students, 4 nursing instructors, 2 academic counselors, and 1 academic administrator. The study is an example of grounded theory methodology using interviews, teacher evaluations, and participant observation. The following categories emerged from the data: "(1) breaking free; (2) coping; acquisition of knowledge and competencies;

(3) stress, coping and support: relationship; (4) coping and learning: support and facilitation; and (5) transitions" (p. 2339). From these categories, propositions were developed. Ultimately, "the substantive theory of adjusting to becoming a nurse was applied to educational practice through developing a curriculum construal and by suggesting uses of the substantive theory for everyday practice" (p. 2339).

Socialization to a role is an important part of successful assimilation into a group. Bradby (1990) uses the process of change to report on the transition of student to nurse. In this study, Bradby followed "four cohorts of female trainee nurses in two schools of nursing" (p. 1221) to discover the reality of the nursing experience for trainee nurses. Data sources included: essays, diaries, and letters to potential recruits, backed-up by self-report questionnaires and psychometric tests for self-esteem and anxiety. Data analysis included coding and developing categories.

Status passage was used as the guiding concept throughout data analysis. The major categories of data reported include: anticipations and entry with sub-concepts of changes, contrasts, and shift rotations; and surprise and reality shock on entering wards. Other sub-concepts of reality shock included: special parts of major status passage; serial passage; disjunctive passage; divestiture; personal identity; collective passage and sense making. The author concludes "the transition into the clinical area may provoke more problems for the student which will continue for some time following completion of the course" (Bradby, 1990, p. 1224).

Student-faculty relationships.   Two studies describe the impact of the student-faculty relationship on socialization of nursing students. Stephenson (1984) conducted a modification of Glaser and Strauss' grounded theory methodology to describe student-faculty relationships. Twenty-two student nurses and 23 nurse tutors were interviewed using a semi-structured interview schedule. Stephenson used study findings to describe the ideal type of tutor-student relationship, which bifurcates into two basic aspects: the teacher-student relationship and the counselor-client relationship. The researcher offers that bureaucratic or professional expectations may impact on the tutor-student relationship.

In a similar study, Kushnir (1986) described stressful interpersonal encounters. In particular, Kushnir was concerned with identifying what impact clinical faculty had on students. Twenty-eight second-year female nursing students were asked to write down an interpersonal encounter which they found stressful. Only 20 encounters were analyzed "since they shared a common kind of stressor" (p. 16). Rather than share type of data analysis, Kushnir did discuss analytic categories developed in four specific areas: type of situation in which the incident occurred; how the stressor behaved in the situation; the respondents' reactions; and the psychological and social-psychological processes which mediated the students' reactions.

Kushnir (1986) states, "the aim of teaching is to reduce errors, especially in critical tasks involving people's lives" (p. 19). The presence of significant others, such as instructors, may increase the error rates of students because of their fear of failure or embarrassment.

Students' retention. Two studies have attempted to gain insight into nursing student role socialization by describing aspects of students' retention. Wilson and Levy (1978) interviewed students who withdrew from an RN completion program to determine why they chose to drop out. The researchers analyzed a theoretical sample of 14 withdrawn students' interviews using grounded theory methodology and identified categories reflective of student withdrawal: difference in how they adjusted, including the themes of matching process and balancing process; and types of withdrawal with the subthemes of stepping out, dropping in, and switching out.

Mashburn (1985) used the case study approach to observe evening/weekend students as they progressed through their diploma program. Two particular areas of interest were the type of nontraditional student and the factors which influenced their progression. Mashburn reports that programmatic factors and personal student factors influenced student progression. Mashburn asserts that study results can be used to develop guidelines for building programs for nontraditional students. Based on the findings, Mashburn identifies the major responsibilities of faculty as representing the program accurately, advising and counseling students, and allowing students to develop personal pathways to learning.

Empathy. Focusing on another aspect of student socialization, Malek (1989) used a combination of quantitative and qualitative methods. Qualitative methods were employed to examine the subjective reality of empathy as perceived by students in their experiences. Eight of 39 students who completed the quantitative measures for the study were interviewed to identify their perceptions of empathy. Analysis of the data revealed specific categories. The conditions students perceive as enhancing their development of empathy include: familiarity/similarity with patients; the experience of having been a patient themselves; verbal communication ability of patients; and illness of a chronic rather than acute nature. The barriers to development of empathy include: age differences; lack of positive reinforcement; time constraints; difficult patients; and fear of death. Malek states that her findings support the perspective that empathy is an evolving process.

Clinical Experience

The lived experience of students in the clinical environment became the major focus of several studies. Windsor (1987) conducted a study via naturalistic inquiry "to better understand the clinical experience from the nursing students' point of view" (p. 150). Nine students enrolled in their final semester of nursing school were interviewed twice. The transcripts were analyzed to identify common categories, including: skill development; time management; professional socialization; preparation; supervision; variety of assignments; personal problems; stages of development; interpersonal relationships; patient care; and need for approval. Windsor (1987) concluded that the value of the study lies in its implications for nursing education and in directions for future research. Specifically, Windsor asserts that few nurses who teach are prepared for this activity. "A better understanding of what constitutes quality clinical education would be valuable in providing better educational experiences" (p. 154). In effect, those who teach should know more about the clinical experience so that they can help students be in those settings. Clinical experience for nursing students is a significant aspect of professional education. "This study reveals many questions which need to be systematically answered [specific to clinical education]" (p. 154).

Two dissertations were found which focused on the area of clinical education. From the student perspective, Byrne (1988) explored "the human experience of learning to the practice of nursing" (p. 2123). The framework for this study was culture and symbolic interactionism. Ethnographic methodology was used to collect and analyze data including student diaries, audiotaped narratives, participant observation, a field journal, and ethnographic interviewing. The participants were 18 nursing students in a generic nursing program.

Study findings reveal that students feel pressured by time, are focused on clinical activities, wish to be valued for their interactions in the clinical setting, experience strong emotions, and find the clinical area extremely unpredictable. Additionally, students recognize the importance of developing observing and listening skills early on in their learning experiences. They also need to feel that they are doing something valuable for patients.

Streubert (1989) in a similar study, sought "to identify what the essences of clinical experience were for nursing students and clinical educators" (p. 906). In her study, phenomenological methodology was used to collect and analyze data from 10 clinical students and faculty. From the analysis, exhaustive descriptions of clinical experience were written for both groups. "Student commentaries were permeated with descriptions of faculty, staff, and patient relations, and feelings related to their role as a student. Faculty verbalized themes reflecting their awareness of responsibility and necessity of acting out a number of different roles (Streubert, 1989, p. 906)." The researcher concludes that it is important for nurse educators and students to know each other if the provision of holistic care is to be facilitated.

Health

Hanna's (1989) study focused on the meaning of health for graduate nursing students. Using the "qualitative descriptive approach of phenomenology . . . to examine the meaning of health for graduate nursing students based on their life experience" (p. 372), Hanna asked 36 graduate nursing students at two schools of nursing to describe in writing a situation in which they experienced a feeling of health. Twenty-nine students returned the descriptions.

Data were analyzed according to the process described by Parse, Coyne, and Smith. From the responses, "68 descriptive expressions were obtained. Of these, 33 reflected an awareness of a physical state and 35 reflected a mental state" (Hanna, 1989, pp. 364–375). The major categories identified under the physical state included ability, appearance, and energy level. Those identified under the mental category included happiness/contentment, anticipation/excitement, and clarity of thinking. A structural definition of health was offered based on the expressive descriptions. Hanna found that graduate students need to be aware of their personal meanings of health. They also must be aware of the meaning of health held by their clients. "The nurse's and the client's meaning of health influence nurse-client interactions related to health care" (p. 375).

Caring

Leininger and Watson (1990) culled a large number of qualitative studies in nursing education from an annual conference on caring. The three studies of concern here focus on the education of students and a description of the caring experience within the context of the student-teacher relationship.

Appleton's (1990) study purported to "describe the meaning of human care and the experience of caring from the perspective of doctoral students during their educational experience in a program of nursing" (p. 79). The author offers that there is "no research addressing the meaning of the experience of caring in academic institutions that offer programs in nursing" (p. 79). From a purposive sample of two doctoral students, the researcher identifies themes related to the "meaning of human care and the lived experience of caring" (p. 79).

Using phenomenological methods of research as described by van Manen and Ray, three significant aspects of caring in nursing education evolved, including: caring as "expressive," a "process," and having an "environmental dimension" (Appleton, 1990, p. 85). Themes emerging from the data related to the expressive aspect were: treating patients with respect; understanding their interdependence; helping them to grow; and letting them become. The themes identified as part of the process of caring included: commitment with subthemes of potential commitment, reciprocal commitment and genuine commitment; caring as involvement, including subthemes of personal, spiritual, holistic, and freedom; and the feeling of belonging or feeling connected that helped informants understand what it is to be human. For this theme, subthemes of reassuring, comforting, knowing, and connected emerged. The environmental aspect of the caring phenomenon included: time to engage in the process of caring and a place that provides support for caring and space. From the researcher's findings, "a model of pedagogical caring was developed to augment the understanding of caring as a whole" (p. 92). Appleton also proposed that an ontology of compassion creates "caring relationships, situations and academic environments" (p. 92).

Halldorsdottir (1990) explored "the phenomena of caring and uncaring in nursing education, as perceived by former students, so as to know and understand these phenomena more fully" (p. 96). Although Halldorsdottir did not identify a specific study method, the author does describe the process for carrying out the study which includes the use of theoretical sampling, intensive unstructured interviews, and the use of constant comparative analysis. Informants were nine former nursing students, four with BSN degrees, four with MSN degrees and one PhD student.

The study findings reveal that four basic components are part of "the essential structure of a caring encounter with a teacher from the student's perspective" (Halldorsdottir, 1990, p. 97). These include: "the teacher's professional caring approach; the resulting mutual trust and professional teacher-student working relationship; and finally the positive student responses to the caring encounter" (p. 97). The four basic components of an uncaring encounter are "the teacher's lack of professional caring; the resulting lack of trust; teacher-student detachment; and negative student responses to the uncaring encounter" (p. 102).

Halldorsdottir (1990) offers subthemes for many components of caring and uncaring encounters and concludes that such studies "offer hope for increased caring and decreased uncaring in . . . future care providers' learning experiences" (p. 105).

In a similar study, Miller, Haber, and Byrne (1990) were interested in adding "to the understanding of the phenomenon of educational caring by asking students and teachers to recall and describe an interaction involving caring in the teaching-learning process" (p. 126). The researchers used the methods "developed by Streubert and adapted from the works of Colaizzi, Giorgi, Valle, and King" (p. 126).

Informants were a "convenience and purposive sample of six senior nursing students and six nursing faculty" (Miller, Haber, & Byrne, 1990, p. 127). One transcript was unusable, resulting in 11 transcripts for analysis. The four major themes resulting from analysis of both the faculty and student transcripts were: "holistic concern or philosophy; teacher ways of being; mutual simultaneous dimensions; and student ways of being" (p. 128). In this report, the researchers included exhaustive descriptions for both students and faculty. The researchers conclude "students and faculty [describe] caring as a crucial dimension of the education phenomenon [suggesting] that caring as a curriculum foundation or thread should be more fully and clearly developed in nursing programs" (p. 132).

In a study reported by Klisch (1990), the caring theme moves from the academic environment to the practice arena. Klisch states that the purpose of the study "was to identify common reactions of nursing students to their first experience of giving care to a person who is HIV positive" (p. 17). Data were collected via semi-structured interviews with eleven nursing students. The researcher reports that student "reactions were analyzed using a qualitative methodology based on the four phases of the nurse-patient relationship" (p. 16). The pre-interaction phase of the nurse-patient relationship was characterized by anxiety related to fear of the unknown, lack of knowledge about what to do or say while caring for the patient, an inability to relax, and general feelings of discomfort.

In the introductory phase, students "most common reaction was fear, followed by compensatory measures to deal with fear" (Klisch, 1990, p. 17). The fear expressed by students was related to their fear of exposure. During the working phase, students' reactions were characterized by the movement toward meeting the clients' needs and identification with the patient for whom they were caring. In the termination phase, student reactions were characterized by their feelings of closeness to the patient.

Klisch (1990) reports that students have strong emotional responses to caring for individuals infected with AIDS. Although students receive theoretical content, they are unprepared for the reality of the experience of caring for these individuals. While the students are faced with a number of anxieties including those related to their own lifestyles, they perceived that caring for an AIDS infected individual is a growth experience and that all students should have the opportunity.

Based on her findings, Klisch (1990) recommends "faculty should be aware of the needs of students who will be caring for a person with AIDS for the first time" (p. 19). After the caregiving experience, faculty should provide students with the opportunity to discuss their feelings.

FACULTY

Several research studies have been conducted to gain an understanding of faculty experience of the nurse educator role. Unfortunately, only one of these studies has been published. Because the remaining unpublished studies have been conducted as doctoral dissertations, this review is based mainly on published abstracts of those studies. Of the studies completed, three have used phenomenological methodology to describe facets of the faculty role, including: role conflict, response to change, and the role itself.

Role Conflict

Pappas (1988) sought to clarify and describe faculty role conflict using a phenomenological research approach. She postulated that role conflict existed in nursing faculty because of the multiple role expectations of teaching, service, research, and practice. Pappas interviewed 16 baccalaureate nursing faculty to determine perceptions of their multifaceted roles, their experiences of role conflict, their coping strategies, and their feelings of "professional role success or disappointment" (p. 4234).

Pappas (1988) analyzed the transcripts for emergent themes and patterns and for "atypicality" (p. 4234). Although the experience of role conflict was unique for each faculty participant, common patterns emerged from the descriptions. Pappas identified nine categories of professional role conflict. In addition, Pappas described two patterns of role expectation for tenured and non-tenured faculty. Recurring themes of ethical and monetary issues emerged as affecting role conflict and coping. Coping strategies of faculty were described as "a combination of cognitive and emotion-focused strategies and emphasized personal prioritizing" (p. 4243). A desire for a mentoring system also was a recurring theme.

Response to Change

Similarly, Davis (1991) used a phenomenological approach and new paradigm research methodology developed by Reason and Rowan to gain an understanding of the meaning of change to individuals in the academic setting. Subjects included 21 student nurses, 34 faculty, and 11 support staff. The study began with a mailed questionnaire that was designed with open-ended questions to elicit subjects' thoughts and feelings about change. Subjects' responses to the initial questionnaires were analyzed and grouped into categories. Using the Delphi technique, further questionnaires based on the original responses were mailed to subjects. Finally, six of the original 76 subjects were interviewed in depth to gain a deeper understanding of the meaning of change.

Two patterns of behavior in response to change—active and passive participants in change—emerged from the data. A pervasive theme emerged, the concept of "good change" (Davis, 1991, p. 113), that was characterized by a partnership between participants, manager and student, or student and teacher. When a good change occurs, the relationship in this partnership is "open, supportive, and trusting" (p. 113). Davis found that in the nursing changes studied a good change relationship often was absent. Davis also noted the crucial influence of the relationship between those individuals at the top and those individuals at the bottom of the hierarchy in change. A greater demarcation between the top and the bottom is associated with more resistance to change. Davis suggests further study of the partnership relationship during change for future studies.

Faculty Role

Four facets of the faculty role have been studied: faculty practice; research; clinical teaching; and joint appointment.

Faculty practice. Durand (1985) interviewed 20 nurses to "explore the meaning of faculty practice to nurse faculty, clinical specialists, and doctoral students, and [to] examine relationships between practice and theory in the context of faculty and nursing's social mission" (p. 3782). The research method was both phenomenological and participatory. Using phenomenological methodology for analysis and Habermas' critical theory as a framework, Durand presents participants' descriptions and concludes that those descriptions reflect "current [nursing] theory and research are largely irrelevant to [nursing] practice" (p. 3782). Based on participant data, she describes curricula as lacking "pertinence to realities of practice" (p. 3782). She also describes nursing faculty as having an "intellectual rather than personal commitment to practice" (p. 3782). Conceptualization of faculty practice and its importance also differed widely among participants. Durand describes this lack of consensus as detrimental to nursing education and to the nursing profession.

In conclusion, Durand (1985) suggests that critical theory might be used as a framework to create innovative ways of conceptualizing theory, practice, and research. She says, "nursing's knowledge base must be reexamined in light of nursing's interest; cultural unity between the education and practice arms of the profession must be restored; the nature of curriculum and the relationship of faculty to theory and practice must be transformed" (p. 3782).

Faculty Research

Kearney (1987) has studied an additional facet of the nurse faculty role; how nurse researchers "produce and reproduce knowledge for the discipline, identify individual and environmental variables related to successful research outcomes, and generate a theoretical model for research productivity" (p. 2263). Using naturalistic inquiry and an organization systems framework, Kearney interviewed 21 successful nurse faculty researchers at seven of the top ten colleges of nursing. Transcripts of interviews were analyzed using an ethnographic approach for domains and themes.

> From the interviews, the following significant individual variables were identified for the model of research productivity: character traits (interest, commitment and motivation, perseverance, creativity, independence, ethics); knowledge (knowledge base, opportunities for learning, awareness of when consultation and collaboration was appropriate); and skills (mental abilities, interpersonal skills, organizational skills, articulation skills) (p. 2263).

Environmental variables described in the model included: "academic and disciplinary expectations for scholarly productivity; administrative support for nurse faculty's development and involvement in programs of research through workload allocations; provision of resources for environments that capitalize on resources available in academic nursing programs; and collegial support" (p. 2263).

Kearney (1987) suggests further empirical testing of her model of research productivity as applied to academic nursing programs. She also suggests research comparing the research productivity of nurse researchers in clinical settings to those in academic settings.

Clinical teaching. Several nurse education researchers have used case study methodology to describe the faculty clinical instruction role including faculty/clinical joint appointments. Ress (1986) began her study by first logging her own daily instructional activities, which resulted in the identification of 25 clinical nursing instructional activities. These activities included four categories:

"client assignment; group activities; peer activities; and one to one interaction" (p. 1491).

Ress (1986) then developed a "valuation and utility" scale (p. 1491) to provide for faculty ranking of perceived value and capability of using each of the activities in the clinical setting. Using structured observation, logs of instructional activities, interview of nursing faculty implementing the clinical teaching role, and student completed questionnaires, Ress gathered data from active participants in clinical education. Her purpose was to develop a "model of clinical nursing instruction" (p. 1491).

From analysis of data gathered, Ress (1986) developed "The Need Identification-Fulfillment Model of Clinical Nursing Instruction" (p. 1491). The model contained a description of participants, their goals, the environment, instructional processes, and their effects. A theme throughout the observation was importance of the faculty-student group interaction in the clinical teaching process.

Kinney (1985) sought to further describe the faculty role in clinical education in a case study designed to "explore the manner in which faculty members verbally and nonverbally structure clinical laboratory experiences in order to make overt the relationships between theory and practice" (p. 1117). Kinney observed and interviewed students and one faculty member in one clinical experience to describe faculty strategies utilized to articulate theory and practice in the clinical setting. Analysis of the data revealed that clinical assignments were insufficient in articulating theory with practice in the clinical setting. The faculty member supplemented the clinical assignment with "verbal structuring" (p. 1117) and the student completed independent learning activities to achieve theory-practice articulation. In addition, student peers often assist each other in the application of theory to practice.

Theory articulation with practice in clinical teaching also was the subject of Wickenden's (1988) study. Wickenden implemented a self-directed learning program in the clinical education of nursing students in two clinical settings. Her research consists of a case study evaluation of the program. The implementation of the program was described from the student, staff nurse, and clinical faculty perspective.

Findings from the study demonstrate that although the planning and production of learning packages which are appropriate for use in clinical areas is both time-consuming and initially expensive, their use in promoting learning and in helping "students form a wide range of educational abilities to apply theory to practice is effective" (Wickenden, 1988, p. 3112). Recurring themes throughout the case study were the need for a "partnership approach" (p. 3112) between faculty and nursing staff in the clinical teaching situation and the need for flexibility in the faculty member to accommodate to the ever-changing faculty role when self-directed learning approaches are used.

   Joint appointment.   Hoffart (1989) completed a study designed to "provide an increased understanding of the joint appointment position . . . of joint appointees in nursing organizations" (p. 4453). Using interview technique, Hoffart describes the perceptions of eight faculty with a joint clinical appointment to determine how these joint appointees "make sense" (p. 4453) of their roles.

   An in-depth case study presentation of each participant was used to describe the individuality of each sense-making experience. In addition, cross-case analysis resulted in the emergence of themes in sense-making approaches common to all cases. These themes include: "influence of organizational variables on sense-making; temporal aspects of sense-making; approaches for unifying the job; and interactive aspects of sense-making" (Hoffart, 1989, p. 4453). Hoffart notes, however, that the uniqueness of the experiences by far outweigh the similarities. Each participant was able to make sense of the individual experience of joint appointment through these unique sense-making activities.

   Eight studies have been reviewed that principally use nurse faculty as research participants. These studies have provided descriptions of the practice, clinical teaching, research, and joint appointment dimensions of the faculty role; role conflict inherent in the faculty role; and faculty response to change within the academic organization. As a result of two of the studies, models of faculty research productivity and of clinical nursing instruction have been proposed.

   The studies have begun to provide descriptions and understanding of the reality of the human condition of the nurse faculty member. This condition is characterized by a multifaceted role which sometimes results in role conflict. Faculty ability to cope with role conflict and change has been described. Influences on the faculty role include the relationship between faculty members and the principal players in the implementation of their role: their managers, their students, and clinical nurses.

Each of the studies has provided rich data and uncovered areas of concern for further study. Researchers are now faced with the challenge of designing research studies to explore the concerns further.

CURRICULUM

Three nurse education researchers have utilized the case study approach to describe and clarify knowledge of nursing education curriculum. O'Dea (1984) presents a case study of the development of a consortium of associate degree nursing programs and a baccalaureate degree nursing program for the purpose of describing and analyzing the processes involved in its development. The purpose of the consortium was to provide curricular support and enhance career mobility of registered nurse students seeking a baccalaureate degree in nursing.

Data were collected using review of records, surveys and interviews of participants in the development of the consortium. Principles of development of consortia found in the literature were used to analyze the data gathered. Based on analysis of the case study, O'Dea presented guidelines for development of similar consortia and recommended these as guides to developers of nursing educational consortia.

Using published documents and in-depth faculty interviews, Dakin (1987) describes the barriers to faculty implementation of the affective domain in their teaching. The research methodology was a combination of multiple case studies and "collaborative inquiry design" (p. 1002). Five themes emerged from the 13 case studies depicting the barriers to implementing the affective domain: lack of knowledge and experience with the affective domain; the length of time needed to develop affective domain skills in students; the prominence of need for cognitive domain skills dominating curricula; unfamiliarity in interpersonal relationships with students; and a stated recognition of the need for and importance of the affective domain in nursing curricula. Dakin concludes that faculty would benefit from formal education in implementing the affective domain in nursing education.

Diekelmann's (1980) study purported to "analyze textbooks that present the nurse-as-teacher to beginning students by examining how students are introduced to the role of the nurse-as-teacher and what role is presented" (p. 4455). Diekelmann examined five fundamentals of nursing textbooks to describe the conceptualization of the role of the nurse as teacher and students' introduction to this vital role. Using grounded theory to analyze text data, Diekelmann concludes that there is "no existing model for nursing instruction" (p. 4455). She also describes themes common to each of the texts, the most significant being the overall lack of a model of nursing instruction. Authors of each of the texts reviewed have "borrowed" (p. 4455) concepts and principles of teaching and learning from other fields and applied them to nursing without considering either rationally or empirically whether or not these concepts actually apply to the patient-learning situation. A second theme here is an apparent incongruity in the principles of teaching and learning as presented in many texts with a humanistic perspective. Diekelmann concludes that research in patient education specific to nursing is vitally needed. She suggests a number of research questions appropriate for further study.

Nurse educators also have used studies of expert nursing practice to guide curriculum development. Reviewed elsewhere by Tanner (1986) and LeBreck (1989), these studies have been designed using qualitative methodology to describe the essence of expert nursing practice. Pyles and Stern (1983), Phillips and Rempusheski (1985), and Leino-Kilpi (1990) all used a grounded theory approach to describe clinical judgment in critical care nurses, clinical judgment in nurses caring for the elderly, and "good nursing care" (p. 225), respectively. Resulting from these investigations was the development of models of clinical judgment to be used by practicing nurses. Other investigations of expert nurse clinical judgment have used phenomenology as method (Benner 1982, 1984; Brykczynski, 1989; Patterson, 1989). These studies have resulted in a description of the domains of nursing practice and of the common themes influencing nurses' ability to make clinical judgment. Some researchers have suggested that these studies have the potential for guiding nurse educators in curriculum development.

ACADEMIC ADMINISTRATION

Three nursing dissertations have dealt with academic administration. These studies purport to describe an aspect of nursing academic administration and to identify researchable questions which will eventually improve nursing administration practice.

Valentine (1988) and Smith (1987) have used case study methodology to describe aspects of academic administration.

Using behavioral event and critical incident interview schedule, Smith (1987) interviewed four successful nursing school deans to describe the administrative strategies and political skills used by these deans. Smith used a conceptual framework based on "the functional component of strategy found" (p. 695) as described in the literature by the McKinsey 7-S model of excellence. Strategies used by the deans were consistent with those identified in the literature as appropriate for successful organizational leaders. Although the particular strategies used by deans varied, commonalties emerged: variation of strategy used in response to situation, environment, and person; use of both proactive and reactive strategies; and skill in interpersonal relations.

Valentine (1988) used the case study approach to determine if the organizational climate in one school of nursing is characterized by unique orientations to the work place because of the predominance of women in this unique work force. She analyzed the case study within the conceptual framework of "female world" using grounded theory as her analytic approach. The culture of the school and the behavior of the instructors were characteristic of two aspects of the female world described in the literature, Gemeinschaft orientation and love-and/or-duty ethos. Five categories emerged from the data describing the female orientation of the work force: the use of food and social events to create group cohesiveness; the need for each instructor to have a supportive colleague in the work environment; the use of meetings to build group cohesion; the need for cohesiveness and group consensus in dealing with students; and the consistent use of group consensus to make decisions. Valentine fails to make implications for administration practices based on these findings, however.

Using the technique for naturalistic inquiry, Thorpe (1989) interviewed college of nursing administrators to describe the phenomenon of leadership as perceived by these leaders. Three major themes emerged from the seven interviews: "mission or goals; relating to others; and meanings of activities" (p. 4989). Focusing on a specific mission provided meaning for each of the participants. These findings were consistent with those described in the literature by Immegart's model of leadership. Thorpe recommends further interpretative research of nurse academic leadership incorporating followers' perceptions and interpretations into the study.

Although the few studies relating to administration of nursing education have only begun to scratch the surface of the reality of the human condition of nursing education administrators, the descriptions provided thus far are valuable. Yet, researchers need to design additional qualitative studies that describe other areas of concern to nursing education administrators and reveal research questions for further study.

STAFF DEVELOPMENT

Whiteley (1989) used the case study approach to evaluate two continuing education programs of instruction. Although Whiteley fails to identify in the abstract her specific sources of data, she did develop the "Structure-Process-Outcome Model" (p. 4990) for evaluation of continuing education programs based on her techniques. Using progressive functioning and grounded theory techniques, the methodology of evaluation is "predominantly qualitative" (p. 4990). Whiteley proposes that the model is appropriate to guide evaluation of nursing continuation education programs at either the macro or micro level of evaluation.

CONCLUSION

Researchers in nursing education have utilized qualitative research methodologies to understand the reality of nursing education. These studies have addressed student, faculty, curriculum, academic administration, and staff development perspectives of nursing education. Nurse educators have gained insight into the unique experience of being a nursing student in general and specifically in the area of clinical experience, into the unique socialization of the nursing student to student and professional roles, and into the experience of caring from the perspective of the student in both the student-teacher and student-patient relationship. Each of these descriptions provides valuable information for nurse educators in understanding their students. In addition, one qualitative study has been completed to provide both students and their teachers with insight into the student perspective of the meaning of health.

Additionally, qualitative studies have provided nurse educators with insight into the unique role of the nursing faculty member.

The insight includes the areas of faculty practice, research, clinical education, and joint appointment roles. Clarification of the meaning of change and role conflict for faculty members also has been offered.

Nursing education curricular concerns have been elucidated through qualitative inquiry. Completed case studies of curricular innovations provide insight to creators of curriculum change and increase faculty perceptions of the affective domain. Also, studies of expert nurse practice have been completed that have the potential for guiding and influencing curricular innovations. Finally, a few studies provide documentation of insight into academic administration and staff development.

Each of the studies described in this review provides nurse educators with an understanding of the nursing education experience from the unique vision of the participants. A strength of all of the studies is each investigator's success in providing rich descriptive data, including context for the reader's interpretations. This rich data provides readers with the opportunity to identify with areas of mutuality and to begin to understand their own experiences as well as those of others. The questions asked in the studies have been appropriate to qualitative methodologies used and pertinent to the needs of nurse educators. Many researchers reviewed here suggest questions for future research. Yet, this review also suggests that the qualitative research methodologies have not reached their full potential contribution to nursing education. Areas of concern include rigor of method in a number of studies.

Qualitative researchers have developed recognized methods of data gathering, analysis, and trustworthiness in their quest for recognition as rigorous researchers. Most of the studies cited in this review are rigorous in some aspects, but not all. Nearly all the studies identify a recognized method of data gathering. The few that do not (Kinney, 1985; Smith, 1987) can be criticized for lack of rigor and their results questioned.

Many more researchers in the studies cited have failed to identify a recognized format for data analysis in their studies (Bush, 1976; Byrne, 1988; Dakin, 1987; Davis, 1991; Field, 1981; Halldorsdottir, 1990; Kinney, 1985; Malek, 1989; Mashburn, 1985; Massumi, 1989; Nelms, 1990; O'Dea, 1984; Ress, 1986; Smith, 1987; Thorpe, 1989; Wickenden, 1988). Again, failure to identify a recognized method of data analysis lends skepticism to the rigor of the study and its results.

Further skepticism results from the failure of many of the researchers cited to include descriptions of the procedures used for assuring trustworthiness or credibility of the data which early in utilization of qualitative methods was defined as reliability and validity as it applied to qualitative research. Without assurance of trustworthiness and credibility, readers of the report cannot be sure that the descriptions provided accurately represent the perceptions of the participants. Several of the studies reviewed did include this information (Appleton, 1990; Durand, 1985; Hanna, 1989; Kushnir, 1986; Kayser-Jones & Abu-Saad, 1982; Miller, Haber, & Byrne, 1990; Melia, 1982; Ress, 1986; Simms, 1981; Stephenson, 1984; Streubert, 1989; Van Dongen, 1988; Windsor, 1987).

Based on the fact that all of the published research reviewed did not include information which speaks to the three areas of rigor identified, it can be concluded that the rigor of qualitative research in nursing education is in its infancy. To provide the most meaningful descriptions of nursing education, studies should clearly follow established procedure for data collection, data analysis, and assurance of trustworthiness. Assurance of rigor will provide meaningful descriptions that will more effectively increase our understanding of the human condition of nursing education.

One can observe that there are far fewer qualitative studies published in the nursing literature than quantitative studies. The questions that arise from this observation are: Are education researchers reluctant to use qualitative research methodologies?; or, Are editors of nursing journals and editorial boards receiving less qualitative manuscripts?; or, Are the qualitative manuscripts which are received not meeting the expectations set by the journals?

An explanation for the paucity of published education research using qualitative methods may be grounded in the nursing profession's desire for recognition as a scientific profession resulting in adoption of the predominant research paradigm. Nurses as a group have relied on other recognized professions to guide their research methods, especially the quantitative methodologies of the medical profession (Watson, 1981; Melia, 1982).

A second explanation may be the lack of experienced qualitative researchers to entice prospective researchers or to act as their mentors. The question arises whether nursing students are introduced to philosophy of science and the nature of inquiry in all of its dimensions before they are introduced to research methodology. The result is student development of projects or the critique of experts' words based on an inadequate and at times inaccurate perception of the nature of inquiry.

An issue which arises from this critique is the methodological application and reporting of qualitative research. We would suggest that part of the concern with the methodologies used in this review is that many of them have been reported without speaking to the purpose of the method or the reason for deviation from methods adopted from psychology, philosophy, anthropology, and education. This may be a direct result of reporting qualitative findings in journals which have traditionally published quantitative studies in 12 to 15 pages. Or, it may be a result of the researcher's lack of expertise with the method or the neophyte nature of qualitative research in the discipline. For example, the expected outcome of using grounded theory is the generation of a formal or substantive theory (Hutchinson, 1986). In many cases in this review, grounded theory methods of data analysis have been employed without generation of a testable theory as Glaser and Strauss (1967) originally intended.

FUTURE DIRECTIONS

The use of qualitative research methodologies is in its infancy in the nursing profession in general and in nursing education specifically. The nature of qualitative research is consistent with nurses' ways of being in clinical practice. This makes it appealing to those who are philosophically committed to interact with research as a way of being. Nurses who have been introduced to qualitative research often are grounded in its underlying philosophy, and thus, the congruency between this research philosophy and the philosophy of nursing. The congruency of method and philosophy attracts neophyte researchers to qualitative methodology. The attraction creates its own challenges because those who are introduced to the method may not fully understand the complexity of implementing it. The responsibility of the profession is to view the research which has been published recognizing its infancy and maintain a critical perspective toward what can be.

Qualitative methods described in this review in many instances have been used appropriately to describe faculty and student experiences of their educational journeys. Even those studies which have required the reader to give the researcher a greater latitude in the interpretation of their data without more guidance as to their method or procedures has shared an important understanding of the participants' experiences. This understanding will provide new insight into the condition of nursing education.

REFERENCES

Appleton, C. (1990). The meaning of human care and the experience of caring in a university school of nursing. In M. M. Leininger & J. Watson (Eds.), *The caring imperative in nursing education* (pp. 77–94), New York: National League for Nursing.

Benner, P. (1982). From novice to expert. *American Journal of Nursing, 82,* 23–31.

Benner, P. (1984). *From novice to expert.* Menlo Park, CA: Addison Wesley.

Brykczynski, K. (1989). An interpretative study describing the clinical judgment of nurse practitioners. *Scholarly Inquiry for Nursing Practice: An International Journal, 3,* 75–103.

Bush, P. J. (1976). The male nurse: A challenge to traditional role identities. *Nursing Forum, 15,* 390–405.

Bradby, M. (1990). Status passage into nursing: Another view of the process of socialization in nursing. *Journal of Advanced Nursing, 15,* 1220–1225.

Byrne, M. W. (1988). An ethnography of undergraduate nursing students' clinical learning field. *Dissertation Abstracts International, 49,* 2123.

Dakin, C. (1987). Affective curriculum in nursing education: A case study of the intrinsic and extrinsic barriers experienced by nurse educators in the implementation process. *Dissertation Abstracts International, 48,* 1002.

Davis, P. (1991). The meaning of change to individuals within a college of nurse education. *Journal of Advanced Nursing, 16,* 108–115.

Diekelmann, N. (1980). The nurse-as-teacher: An analysis of fundamentals of nursing textbooks. *Dissertation Abstracts International, 41,* 4455.

Durand, B. (1985). The relationship of practice and theory in the context of nursing faculty. *Dissertation Abstracts International, 46,* 3782.

Field, P. A. (1981). A phenomenological look at giving an injection. *Journal of Advanced Nursing, 6,* 291–296.

Glaser, B. G., & Strauss, A. L. (1967). *The discovery of grounded theory.* Chicago: Aldine.

Grassi-Russo, N., & Morris, P. B. (1981). Hopes and fears: The attitudes of freshmen nursing students. *Journal of Nursing Education, 20*(6), 9–17.

Halldorsdottir, S. (1990). The essential structure of caring and uncaring encounter with a teacher: The perspective of the nursing student. In M. M. Leininger & J. Watson (Eds.), *The caring imperative in nursing education* (pp. 95–108). New York: National League for Nursing.

Hanna, K. M. (1989). The meaning of health for graduate nursing students. *Journal of Nursing Education, 28,* 372–376.

Hoffart, N. (1989). Organizational sense-making by nursing joint appointees. *Dissertation Abstracts International, 50,* 4453.

Hutchinson, S. (1986). Grounded theory: The method. In P. Munhall & C. Oiler (Eds.) *Nursing Research: A qualitative perspective* (pp. 3–26), Norwalk, CT: Appleton-Century-Crofts.

Kayser-Jones, J. S., & Abu-Saad, H. (1982). Loneliness: Its relationship to the educational experience of international nursing students in the United States. *Western Journal of Nursing Research, 4,* 301–315.

Kearney, R. (1987). A model for nurse faculty research productivity. *Dissertation Abstracts International, 48,* 2263.

Kinney, R. (1985). Relating theoretical and clinical content in nursing: A qualitative case study. *Dissertation Abstracts International, 46,* 1117.

Klisch, M. L. (1990). Caring for persons with AIDS: Student reactions. *Nurse Educator, 14,* 16–20.

Kushnir, T. (1986). Stress and social facilitation: The effects of the presence of an instructor on student nurses' behavior. *Journal of Advanced Nursing, 11,* 13–19.

LeBreck, D. (1989). Clinical judgement: A comparison of theoretical perspectives. In W. Holzemer (Ed.), *Review of Research in*

Nursing Education (Vol. II) (pp. 33–35), New York: National League for Nursing.

Leininger, M. M., & Watson, J. (1990). *The caring imperative in education.* New York: National League for Nursing.

Leino-Kilpi, H. (1990). Good nursing care: On what basis? *Dissertation Abstracts International, 51,* 255.

Malek, C. J. (1989). The socialization of empathy: A study of neophyte baccalaureate student nurses. *Dissertation Abstracts International, 50,* 2846.

Mashburn, P. A. (1985). Nontraditional nursing students in a part-time evening/weekend diploma program. *Dissertation Abstracts International, 50,* 2339.

Massumi, E. M. (1989). Becoming a nurse: Transitions and adjustments. *Dissertation Abstracts International, 50,* 2339.

Melia, K. (1982). "Tell it as it is"—qualitative methodology and nursing research: Understanding the student nurse's world. *Journal of Advanced Nursing, 7,* 321–335.

Miller, B. K., Haber, J., & Byrne, M. (1990). The experience of caring in the teaching-learning process of nursing education: Student and teacher perspectives. In M. M. Leininger & J. Watson (Eds.) *The caring imperative in nursing education* (pp. 1–24), New York: National League for Nursing.

Nelms, T. P. (1990). The lived experience of nursing education: A phenomenological study. In M. M. Leininger & J. Watson (Eds.), *The caring imperative in nursing education* (pp. 285–297), New York: National League for Nursing.

O'Dea, E. (1984). Description and critical analysis of the processes related to the development of a nursing education consortium. *Dissertation Abstracts International, 45,* 2498.

Olsen, B., & Whittaker, F. (1968). *The silent dialogue.* San Francisco: Jossey-Bass.

Pappas, A. (1988). Professional role conflict and related coping strategies of baccalaureate nursing faculty: A phenomenological study. *Dissertation Abstracts International, 49,* 4234.

Patterson, R. (1989). Domains of nursing practice: Application of Benner's model. *Dissertation Abstracts International, 50,* 5550.

Phillips, L., & Rampusheski, V. (1985). A decision-making model for diagnosing and intervening in elder abuse and neglect. *Nursing Research, 34,* 134–139.

Pyles, S., & Stern, P. (1983). Discovery of nursing gestalt in critical care nursing: The importance of the gray gorilla syndrome. *Image: The Journal of Nursing Scholarship, 15,* 51–57.

Ress, M. (1986). An elucidation of a model of clinical nursing instruction from actual clinical nursing instructional practice. *Dissertation Abstracts International, 47,* 1491.

Simms, L. M. (1981). The grounded theory approach in nursing. *Nursing Research, 30,* 356–359.

Smith, D. (1987). The strategies and political skills used by successful nursing deans: A descriptive study, *Dissertation Abstracts International, 49,* 696.

Stephenson, P. M. (1984). Aspects of the nurse tutor-student nurse relationship. *Journal of Advanced Nursing, 9,* 283–290.

Streubert, H. J. (1979). A description of clinical experience as perceived by clinical nursing educators and students. *Dissertation Abstracts International, 50,* 906.

Tanner, C. (1986). Research on clinical judgment. In W. Holzemer (Ed.) *Review of research in nursing education* (Vol. I) (pp. 3–40), New York: The National League for Nursing.

Thorpe, K. (1989). Interpreting the activities of nursing educational administrators: A leadership perspective, *Dissertation Abstracts International, 50,* 4989.

Valentine, P. (1988). A hospital school of nursing: A case study of a predominantly female organization, *Dissertation Abstracts International, 49,* 4238.

Van Dongen, C. J. (1988). The life experience of the first-year doctoral student. *Nurse Educator, 13,* 19–24.

Watson, J. (1986). Nursing's scientific quest. *Nursing Outlook,* 413–416.

Whiteley, S. (1989). The construction of an evaluation model for use in conjunction with continuing education courses in the nursing profession. *Dissertation Abstracts International, 50,* 4990.

Wickenden, S. (1988). Self-directed learning in nurse education: A case study on an orthopaedic ward. *Dissertation Abstracts International, 49,* 3112.

Wilson, H. S., & Levy, J. (1978). Why RN students drop out. *Nursing Outlook, 26,* 437–441.

Windsor, A. (1987). Nursing students' perceptions of experience. *Journal of Nursing Education, 26,* 150–154.

Chapter Four

NURSING RESEARCH RELATED TO EDUCATIONAL RE-ENTRY FOR THE REGISTERED NURSE

Cecile Lengacher, PhD, RN
Mary Lou VanCott, PhD, RN

Emphasizing the baccalaureate in nursing as the entrance degree for professional nursing practice, university based nursing schools now face an increasing enrollment of students who are licensed nurses (RN students). As a result, nurse educators are encountering the problems of how to address the varied needs and issues of these special, nontraditional students. This chapter includes a review of current research related to educational re-entry for the registered nurse.

REGISTERED NURSE EDUCATION: SIGNIFICANCE FOR RESEARCH

Despite intense efforts to attract students to generic nursing programs, the largest portion, some 66.5 percent, of American nurses are prepared at either the diploma and the associate degree levels (NLN, 1991). The importance of research on this population re-entering the educational arena becomes obvious when considering that the majority of registered nurses practicing today do not have baccalaureate degrees. During the past ten years, baccalaureate graduations from basic programs are reported to have decreased 11.6 percent while the number of RNs graduating from baccalaureate programs has increased from 9,594 in 1985 to 11,546 in 1989 (NLN, 1991). Nonbaccalaureate prepared registered nurses, motivated by a variety of personal and professional reasons, are enrolling in baccalaureate programs to complete their degrees. The need for nurses with additional educational credentials has dramatically increased within the health care system (USDHHS, 1988). Nurse educators are then confronted with issues related to access to the baccalaureate in nursing for the RN

75

student population and the need to develop curricular options which will enhance the student's progression through the education process.

The need for access to institutions of higher education is particularly difficult for registered nurses who are unable to enroll in baccalaureate programs due to employment and/or family responsibilities, or those who are located in remote geographical areas. Historically, mobility programs for RNs have been slow to develop primarily due to lack of available resources, issues of validation of prior learning, and issues of accreditation. While growth in programs has been slow, recently there has been an increase in the number of registered nurse students seeking admission into baccalaureate programs.

More RNs than ever are seeking and demanding an education beyond their basic associate degree or diploma in nursing. There has been a reported increase of associate degree graduates seeking a baccalaureate degree in the past five years from 5,479 in 1985 to 7,194 in 1989 (NLN, 1991). Many RNs are enrolling in programs because they are personally motivated to achieve a higher educational level as a measure of their own success. Colleges and schools of nursing are admitting mature learners who challenge faculty and administration. These students have varied college histories and enter with variable transferable credits and nursing competencies. Nurse faculty in colleges and universities are faced with providing nontraditional and flexible educational experiences while maintaining quality in their programs. In addition, these returning RN students have very different personal and professional histories, ranging from newly graduated to many years of nursing experience. Their age, economic situation, and marital/family status are diverse. In order to assist these students, educational re-entry for RNs has become a focus for nursing research. The analysis of current research, as offered here, will assist educators to improve or change nursing education methodologies and curricula based upon research findings. The need for strong support systems to facilitate the educational success of the RN student has been clearly established.

Definitions and Method

The registered nurse returning to school is viewed here (from 1985 through 1991) as one who is enrolled in or is a potential student to enroll in a program of study at a college or university.

Research articles related to the working RN population not in college were excluded from this study. A computer and manual search was conducted for studies published related to RN student re-entry in the following seven journals: *The Canadian Nurse, Journal of Continuing Education in Nursing, Journal of Nursing Education, Journal of Professional Nursing, Nurse Educator, Nursing Research,* and *Western Journal of Nursing Research.* Applicable studies were found in six of the above nursing research journals with the exception of *Nursing Research.* The vast majority of the total 31 studies that were identified as meeting study inclusionary criteria were found in the *Journal of Nursing Education.* Minimum inclusionary criteria included articles that described a scientific research approach that systematically assessed curricular issues or personal characteristics of RN students re-entering the education system to seek a baccalaureate degree. Each study was reviewed related to variables, conceptual frameworks, research design, sampling procedures, data analysis, and research outcomes.

ASSESSMENT OF THE LITERATURE REVIEW

Thirty-one published research investigations related to educational re-entry for RNs were found through a limited review of literature published since 1985. This updated review of nursing research expands upon the work of Dr. Pamela Baj, as published in the 1985 *Review of Research in Nursing Education, Volume I.* The empirical studies included in the present assessment are divided into three major categories for review and discussion: the changing role and role socialization of the RN student; personal characteristics of RN students, which include studies focused on demographic characteristics, developmental patterns, and motivational dimensions; and curricular/programmatic issues including types of programs and innovative teaching/learning strategies specific for use with RN students. A summary of the 31 studies presented in Table 1 shows the clustering of the studies into the three major areas of concern depicted in the literature review. From this summary, it is evident that the most frequently investigated topic (48.4%, n = 15) concerned the description of the personal characteristics of RN students. While eleven studies (35.5%) were concerned with curricular or programmatic issues, the remaining five studies (16.1%) were concerned with the changing role and role socialization of the RN student.

Table 1. Categories of Research Related to Educational Re-entry of the Registered Nurse

Categories	Topics	Researchers	Dates	Sample	Design
Changing role, role socialization	Professionalization	Lawler & Rose	1987	79	Descriptive Ex-post facto
	Role conflict and well-being in multiple role women	Campaniello	1988	155	Descriptive
	Role congruence	Rendon	1988	167	Correlational
	Socialization of RN to BSN	Lynn, McCain, Boss	1989	223	Experimental
	Students' perceptions of roles, effort and performance	Swanson	1987	194	Quasi-experimental
Personal characteristics					
Demographic	Personal characteristic as implications for curriculum	Baj	1985	251	Descriptive
	University challenge	Dugas	1985	364	Analytical survey
	Evolution of baccalaureate program for RNs	MacLean, Knoll & Kinney	1985	198	Retrospective Longitudinal
	Recruiting, advising, and program planning	Lange	1986	965	Descriptive
	Personality characteristics	Everett	1988	51	Longitudinal
	Learning characteristics	Linares	1989	345	Quasi-experimental
	Demographic comparison between on-campus and satellite-center RNs	McClelland & Daly	1991	72	Quasi-experimental
Developmental patterns	Comparison of adult developmental patterns of RNs and Generic students	King	1986	79	Descriptive quasi-experimental

Category	Description	Author	Year	N	Method
	Impact of differences between RNs and Generic students on the educational process	King	1988	79	Descriptive quasi-experimental
	Analyzing coping methods reported by returning RNs	Lee	1988	111	Descriptive
Motivational dimensions	Coping and developmental	Mattson	1990	138	Descriptive
	Recruiting for RN/BSN students	Lange	1986	965	Descriptive
	Motivational dimensions that precipitate return to college	Fotos	1987	57	Descriptive
	Comparison of motivational factors of RNs in two types of programs	Thurber	1988	233	Experimental
	Motivational orientations in rural New England	Lethbridge	1989	132	Descriptive
Curricular and Programmatic Issues					
Types of Programs	RN students in generic programs	Blatchley & Stephen	1985	57	Descriptive
	Locally-based program	Borst & Walker	1986	53	Descriptive
	Extension sites	Tiffany & Burson	1987	30	Descriptive
	Advanced placement policies	Arlton & Miller	1987	238	Descriptive
	Stressful clinical and didactic incidents	Lee	1987	111	Descriptive
	RNs perceptions of their baccalaureate programs	Beeman	1988	284	Quasi-experimental
	Professional resocialization of post-RN baccalaureate students by distance education	Cragg	1991	24	Qualitative

Table 1. (*Continued*)

Categories	Topics	Researchers	Dates	Sample	Design
Innovative Teaching/ Learning Strategies	Changing locus of control with a futuristic-oriented course	DuFault	1985	64	Experimental
	Self-management techniques and the generalization and maintenance of interpersonal skills	Farley & Baker	1987	24	Experimental
	Critical thinking, creativity, clinical performance, achievement	Sullivan	1987	51	Descriptive
	Microcounseling to teach therapeutic communication skills	Daniels, Denny & Andrews	1988	53	Experimental

Of the studies reviewed, the most frequently employed research design (58%) was descriptive/exploratory in nature. Only three of the investigators utilized an experimental method and six used a quasiexperimental design. Only two of the studies had a longitudinal element and there was limited use of time series and no evidence of repeated measures design. Limited use of qualitative research methods, such a phenomenology, ethnography, or grounded theory, was found. There was limited use of multisites for data collection. The studies were highly descriptive.

Few of the studies reviewed were designed to test a theory. While there was evidence of linking of theoretical frameworks to the investigation, most studies were based upon limited, general frameworks of previous research in the area. There was no evidence of commonality in use of theoretical models. This finding is similar to the findings of Stember (1984) who reviewed curricular research in nursing and found that research investigations in the education area were not built upon other studies, either conceptually or methodologically.

DISCUSSION OF CATEGORIES
OF RESEARCH CONCERN

Studies were found in three general areas from the review of published research. In this section, the studies are discussed and examined for their contribution to the knowledge base regarding the returning RN student into baccalaureate education.

The Changing Role and Socialization of RN Students

Research relating to the changing role and role socialization of registered nurse students has been an area of concern in several studies found in education research literature over the past five years (Campaniello, 1988; Lawler & Rose, 1987; Lynn, McCain, & Boss, 1989; Rendon, 1988; Swanson, 1987). Because of the increasingly changing role of women and the profession in contemporary society, this area of research grows more relevant. In this area, studies focused on student role socialization and on potential multiple role conflict experienced by the returning RN student into the academic setting. The five studies in question viewed role conflict from very divergent approaches.

Rendon (1988) examined the degree of congruence between the interpersonal orientation of the RN student seeking a baccalaureate degree in nursing and the student's perception of the student role. This correlational study reviewed role relationships among 167 registered nurse students from five baccalaureate programs. Sixty-six percent were employed on a full-time basis and 33 percent were employed part time. The average age was 30 years, and the average years of nursing experience was five years. The two instruments utilized were the Rendon PSR Scale, which assessed the student's perception of their student role, and the Cohen CAD Scale, which assessed interpersonal orientation.

The Rendon (1988) study suggested that RN students constitute a diverse population but have congruence toward the student role. Results on the PSR scale revealed a strong commitment and determination in the registered nurse student. However, over one-half of the students did not feel respected by their faculty because they were treated as novices while at the same time, perceiving themselves as more clinically competent than their faculty. Correlations were significant between compliant trends and enjoyment/involvement in the student role, and satisfaction with their academic efforts. Students with high aggressive trends showed enjoyment (p < .05) but felt the curriculum was not appropriate (p < .01), and expressed that they were not comfortable with the student role and had little sense of belonging (p < .01). A highly detached orientation was related to believing that the curriculum was not appropriate (p < .01). Findings showed that full-time students had a greater congruence with their student role than part-time students. The perception that the curriculum was less appropriate for the registered nurse increased with the registered nurse's year of experience. Rendon concluded that assertive registered nurse students need to be viewed less critically by educators and considered more as individuals who cope better and will assist in moving the profession forward. Based upon the role characteristics and professional experiences that the learner brings to the academic environment, if faculty are sensitive to role and role congruence, learning could be enhanced. The major strength of this study was the large sample size gathered from five sites.

Campaniello (1988) assessed the effects of multiple roles on professional nurses entering the academic setting. This study examined whether multiple roles increase role conflict; if women with greater social supports exhibited less role conflict than multiple role women with fewer social supports; if sex role concept was related to role conflict and level of well-being; and whether higher perceived role conflict was related to lower well-being. The sample consisted of 155 female students enrolled full time in a baccalaureate program. While a concern in this study is its limitation to one institution, findings do lend important supporting evidence in assisting educators to view students' potential for success in educational programs.

The BEM Inventory (Bem, 1981) classified sex roles as either feminine/undifferentiated or masculine/androgynous and findings showed that 71 percent of respondents held sex role orientations of feminine or undifferentiated, while 29 percent reflected a masculine or androgynous category. The Center for Epidemiological Studies Depression Scale (CES-D) (Radloff, 1977) was used to assess level of well-being. Results showed that employed nurses were not found to experience greater role conflict than nonemployed nurses and no significant differences existed between the means for conflict in married and unmarried women. However, women with children were found to experience significantly greater role conflict than women without children. The most important single variable explaining role conflict was motherhood, and the variable most directly influencing well-being was conflict. In analysis of the CES-D scale, women who had multiple roles experienced greater well-being than those with fewer roles. Parental support services, such as child-care programs and individual group counseling supports, are becoming priorities within academic settings. This research supports the need for such programs within academic settings.

Lawler and Rose (1987) studied the concept of professionalism among 25 senior generic baccalaureate students, 18 senior RN students, and 36 senior associate degree students. This study used an ex-post facto design which compared the differences in professionalism of the three groups of students. Two instruments were used to assess the dimension of professionalism: Stone's Health Care Professional Attitude Inventory (modified by Lawler) and the professional subscale from Corwin's Nursing Role Conception Scale. Results confirmed that there was a difference in nursing graduates prepared at different educational levels with the RN/BSN graduate consistently showing more professional orientation than the generic/BSN or ADN graduate. Lawler and Rose demonstrated that working as an RN could have possibly socialized the nurse to a greater extent than one would expect. The major weakness of this study was the small sample size which limits generalizability of findings. The difference in professionalism between RNs and generic students should be examined further through replication of Lawler and Rose's research.

Lynn, McCain, and Boss (1989) studied professional socialization of the RN to BSN in 30 RN/BSN students and 193 generic BSN students. With the effects of the BSN program on professional socialization examined upon entry and exit, a longitudinal design was utilized. Through use of ANCOVA, RN/BSN students did not demonstrate significant differences from entry to exit on the Nurses' Professional Orientation Scale (NPOS) compared to generic students who did exhibit a significant difference between entry and exit at the .05 level, on socialization scores. The NPOS has demonstrated reliability coefficients of .88 to .92. The Six-Dimension Scale of Nursing Performance (Six-D) was used to supplement the NPOS data upon entry and exit. The Six-D has alpha reliability estimates of .86 to .90. RN/BSN students exhibited higher scores at graduation on the teaching/collaboration, interpersonal/communication, and planning/evaluation scales of the Six-D Scale. In comparing the RN/BSN and generic students, differences upon entry to the program were observed on the NPOS but not upon exit. Upon entering the program, RN/BSN students differed from the generic students on five out of six of the Six-D Scale and, upon exit, they differed only on the professional development scale. Major study strengths included high reliabilities of instruments and the longitudinal design. Major study weaknesses included the small population of RNs and lack of experimental control.

Swanson (1987), in a descriptive study, explored similarities and differences between generic and RN baccalaureate nursing students (N = 194) in total role investment, quality of effort, and nursing performance. Nine nursing programs were used for data collection. The instruments utilized were the Total Role Investment Scale, the Pace College Questionnaire (measured quality of effort), and the Six-Dimension Scale of Nursing Performance modified by Lubno (1984). Through use of an ANOVA, significant differences were found among generic students, generic completion students (RNs) in generic program, and completion RN students. In comparison to the two groups of RN students, generic students were younger and second generation college, predominantly Caucasian, and unmarried. In assessment of total role involvement, RNs, as a group, were significantly higher in their score as compared to generic students (p < .01); however, there were no significant differences between generic completion RN students and completion RN students. There were no significant differences among the three groups of students on total quality of effort, however, total nursing performance was significantly higher for RN generic completion and RN completion students than for generic BSN students. These differences could be taken into account when considering curriculum change. Further considerations for research related to integration of the RN into the student role, role socialization, and professionalism of the RN student should give consideration to larger samples from multiple sites to lend strength to the generalizability of study findings. In addition, examination of working versus nonworking nurses, to determine effects of working on role conflict and well-being, should be addressed. Longitudinal studies could evaluate the direction of the effects of multiple roles upon the registered nurse student.

Personal Characteristics of the RN Student

As nurse educators prepare for providing education for the increasing number of RNs returning to school, the characteristics and special needs of the RN student are a primary concern. These variables will impact upon the RN student's success and satisfaction in baccalaureate education. Fifteen studies were found that concerned personal characteristics of the RN student. The studies reviewed identified three areas of focus and were categorized into: demographic characteristics, developmental patterns, and motivational dimensions of RN students.

Demographic characteristics. The demographic differences between registered nurse students and generic students have been examined in a number of research studies (Baj, 1985; Dugas, 1985; Everett, 1988; Lange, 1986; Linares, 1989; MacLean, Knoll, & Kinney, 1985; McClelland & Daly, 1991). Baj (1985) completed a study of 251 registered nurse and generic students enrolled in the senior year of BSN programs. Baj identified RNS as one of the largest student populations within baccalaureate programs and noted that they were adult learners who brought different characteristics to the classroom. Baj's study offered a unique perspective, including students only from colleges and universities which admitted registered nurses to an NIH-accredited generic baccalaureate program.

Specific demographic variables studied by Baj (1985) indicated distinct differences between the two types of students. Eighty-one percent of generic students as compared to 39.6 percent of registered nurse students were full-time students. There were more married or divorced registered nurses (56.8%) than generic students (34.5%). Registered nurses (13.8%) received less financial aid than generic students (41.5%). Generic students had a higher percentage of marriage or engagements (22.7% vs. 11.3%) but fewer childbirths compared to registered nurses (9.2% vs. .9%). The registered nurse student also had a higher incidence of family illness (14.2% vs. 7.3%). An unexpected finding was that both groups had one or more dependents. Registered nurses were older (M = 32) than generic students (M = 23) and employed more hours in nursing (27 hours per week compared to 11.49 hours), resulting in a monthly household income for registered nurses of $2,150 compared to $1,630 for generic students.

Specific questions concerning registered nurses showed that 51 percent had been a registered nurse for six or more years. The majority (81.6%) worked in acute care settings, 61.7 percent were employed in medical/surgical areas, and 55.3 percent of the number in acute care worked as staff nurses. One-third of all registered nurses held positions as either assistant head nurses or head nurses. The major strengths of this study were the large sample size and multiple data collection sites utilized.

McClelland and Daly (1991) compared two groups of RN students (N = 72) on demographic characteristics and academic performance. Differences between the on-campus RN student and the satellite campus RN student revealed that students at satellite centers were older, employed, worked more hours per week, traveled farther to class, had more children, and planned on a longer time in which to complete their studies than RNs on the main campus. In performance, satellite-campus RNs had higher ACT-PEP mean scores and transfer GPAs than RNs on campus. Using an analysis of covariance, significant differences were found on grades in two courses: grades for satellite campus students were lower than those for on-campus RN students, but satellite campus RNs worked more, had more children, and drove further to class. Major study limitations included the small sample size and the comparison of grades in only two courses.

In comparison, MacLean, Knoll, and Kinney (1985) examined the graduates (N = 198) of an RN/BSN program in a longitudinal study over an eight-year period. Data collected were descriptive and identified demographic variables, type of programs originally graduated from, length of program, and related variable and effectiveness of the program. Findings showed that, in 1972, 9 percent of students were single as compared to 70 percent in 1978. In addition, length of time in the program decreased between 1971 from an average of 6.6 years to 4.3 years in 1979. Professional activity increased after graduation to 59 percent as compared to 47 percent prior to enrollment in the program. A major limitation of this data is that it is dated but it does give a retrospective perspective for researchers who plan to evaluate RN/BSN programs.

Everett (1988) conducted a longitudinal study to identify specific personality characteristics of RNs returning for their baccalaureate degree. The intent of the evaluation was to use the data to individualize the baccalaureate program to the special needs of the RN student. The sample consisted of two groups for comparison: 31 RN baccalaureate degree students and 20 diploma school students. The study assessed differences in personality characteristics as measured by the California Psychological Inventory. Results indicated that although many RN students had graduated from a diploma program, they demonstrated the qualities and values of individuals from generic baccalaureate programs, and the diploma students demonstrated more traditional characteristics. Results indicated that RN students were characterized as "mature, forceful, strong, aggressive, and independent with leadership potential, and superior intellectual ability." Furthermore, RNs appear more respectful and accepting of others, appreciative, helpful, gentle, conscientious, and sympathetic than the diploma school students. Diploma students, on the other hand, were characterized as more impatient, manipulative, inhibited and unsure, and more likely to act submissively and to comply with authority. Major study weakness included the small sample size. Despite this weakness, Everett's study does suggest that curricula should focus on developing characteristics consistent with the behaviors expected in the profession: leadership, accountability, responsibility, and scholarly inquiry. Future studies could focus on developing characteristics consistent with professional behaviors.

Linares (1989) examined differences in learning characteristics (constructs of locus of control, self-directed learning readiness, and learning style preference) between 170 RNs and 175 generic students. Three instruments were used to assess the constructs: the Adult Nowicki Strickland Internal-External Scale, the Learning Preference Inventory, and the Self-Directed Learning

Readiness Scale. Sample characteristics included the facts that 75.9 percent of the RNs had received an associate degree in nursing and that the majority of RNs had held their credential for more than five years. The majority were employed in acute care settings. These characteristics are consistent with the study by Baj (1985). The sample was attained by volunteers in the first nursing course of the program. The methodology appeared to be a quasiexperimental design.

The research hypothesis that there would be significant differences in self-directed learning and learning style preferences, and locus of control between RN and generic students was not supported. Results did suggest that nursing students had a lower mean score (internal locus of control) than previously reported college students and that nursing students were more self-directed in their learning as compared to a general large sample of adults. Linares reported, however, that statistically significant differences were found among ethnic groups for locus of control; for example, Caucasian students were more internal in their locus of control than black or Hispanic students. Also, Linares reported that Hispanic students scored lower than black or Caucasian subjects on the Self-Directed Learning Readiness Scale. Hispanic and black students indicated a greater preference for the concrete learning mode than Caucasian subjects. Age appeared to influence readiness with older students showing a greater readiness than younger students. Although Linares is to be commended for the large sample size in the study, caution should be taken in interpretation of the results due to a lack of reporting on reliability and validity of the instruments used for data collection. Linares' study also indicated an area requiring further study: the learning needs of individuals with differing ethnicity. Having received very limited study within the RN student population, the learning needs of individuals with differing ethnicity reveals an area for further research.

Lange (1986) conducted a study which has significant implications for recruitment and advisement of registered nurse students. This study surveyed 965 RNs for the purpose of identifying the level of interest and plans to enroll in baccalaureate nursing education, in order to obtain data for recruiting, advising, and program planning for RN/BSN students. Results showed that there were significant differences between respondents who were very interested and those who were not interested in a BSN on certain characteristics such as marital status, age, year of graduation from their basic program, and reasons for obtaining a BSN. This study found that those who planned to enroll were younger, less likely to be married, more likely to hold associate degrees, and to have graduated more recently. Lange recommended advisement conferences be held to discuss lifestyle changes which could facilitate the new role of student. A major study strength included the large sample size.

In a similar study, Dugas (1985) surveyed a random sample of 364 Canadian registered nurses for the purpose of identifying the number, characteristics, interest in returning for a baccalaureate, and needs related to desired courses and scheduling and location of courses. Dugas was primarily concerned about delivery of courses over a teleconference mode which, in Canada, has proven to be quite successful. The method used for the study was an analytical survey. Seventy-five percent of the sample graduated from a diploma program in nursing. One-third of these said they had taken some university courses in the past ten years and were interested in continuing their education. Ninety-three percent indicated an interest in credit courses in the areas of administration, public health, and teaching, and 70.5 percent preferred evening classes. The preferred method of instruction was identified as classroom teaching (97.3%), 36.2 percent for correspondence courses, and 19.5 percent for televised courses. The nurses sampled indicated they wanted continuing education courses which carried credit toward a baccalaureate degree. The primary barrier to further education was identified as family responsibilities.

Developmental patterns. King (1986, 1988), Mattson (1990), and Lee (1988) all focused on developmental patterns of RN students. As identified from the previously reviewed studies, RN students come into the educational system with multiple roles and responsibilities. Their level of developmental maturity could have potential impact on their educational experience. King (1986) conducted a descriptive comparative study designed to identify significant developmental differences on the variables of life stages, ego development, and learning styles. This study used a conceptual framework by Weathersby which incorporates the life stages as defined by Levinson (1978), ego development as defined by Loevinger (1976), and learning styles theories as defined by Kolb (1974).

The sample consisted of 49 registered nurses and 30 generic senior students of one program. Three instruments were used to assess developmental patterns: the Washington University Sentence Completion Test (WUSC) (Loevinger & Wessler, 1970) which measured ego development; the Kolb Learning Style Inventory (Kolb, 1974) which assessed learning styles (divergers, convergers, assimilators, or accommodators), and the Tarule's Education Experience Inventory by Weathersby (1977) which measured life phases and the impact of education on adult development. Results showed that registered nurses and generic students differed on the demographic variables of age, number of semesters completed in school, previous attendance at other institutions, previous degrees, and marital status. Results showed significant differences among the groups in relationship to life stage and ego development. The majority of generic students (83.3%) were in Early Adult Transition, while the majority (36.5%) of registered nurses were in Age 30 Transition or Mid-Life Transition (18.3%). This indicated that the RN student had already made choices about life (marriage, family, love, peers). Early Adult Transition for generic students meant they were beginning to form adult identities with an emphasis on self-discovery.

In the comparison of RNs and generic students on ego development, RNs scored significantly ($p < .05$) higher than generic students. Registered nurse students perceived their education as an investment for the future and as a lifelong process, whereas generic students perceived their education primarily as a future investment.

In assessment of learning styles, the differences between RN and generic students were not significant. Seventy-five percent of both groups of students were categorized as divergers or accommodators. King (1986) described divergers to use "concrete experience and reflective observation" and divergers as proficient at the use of "concrete experience and active experimentation" (p. 367). King proposed that the similarities in RN and generic students' learning styles may be explained by Wolfe and Kolb's (1979) theory that particular professions attract certain types of learners.

In a follow-up study, King (1988) compared 49 registered nurse students to 30 generic students on adult development, student development, and program characteristics valued, while also looking at the impact on the educational process per se. Findings indicated that RNs and traditional students differed significantly in ego development and life stage, but not on learning style. According to King, RNs scored significantly ($p = .05$) higher in ego development (M = 182.88 versus M = 173.92) than generic students. King suggested that "the RNs perceptions, conceptualizations, and interpretations of life events were more advanced than the generic students" (p. 132). The two groups also differed on perception of program characteristics. RNs felt they had more flexibility, autonomy, and independent goal setting as compared to generic students who felt they had less autonomy, flexibility, and independence in goal setting. In this regard, the dual track curricula model could be an effective strategy to help facilitate adult development needs of RN students. The RN students had higher education program satisfaction scores. Life stage appears to have implications for curricular design. King believes that curricular design should be sensitive to developmental needs of students. The major study limitation included the small sample size.

Using the theoretical frameworking of Lazarus, Lee (1988) studied coping methods reported by returning registered nurses. Similarities and differences in RNs between programs designed to integrate the RN into a generic program and those specially designed for the registered nurse were discussed. The study sample consisted of 111 students, 71 of which were enrolled in a specially designed program for RNs, with the remaining 40 enrolled in a generic program.

A critical incident technique questionnaire was used for data collection. Students were asked to describe how they coped with a stressful situation in the classroom and in a clinical situation. Coping strategies were categorized as direct action, such as verbal response, social networking, preparation against harm, avoidance, attack and inaction, or as palliation such as intrapsychic coping or somatic coping. Findings revealed coping methods for students in each program were similar in that 82 percent of respondents used direct action with 58 percent of the responses involving preparation against harm and social networking. Palliation was a method used for only 18 percent of responses. The findings of this study are limited in generalizability due to the small sample size and the convenience sampling.

In an attempt to identify factors useful in predicting effective coping in the RN student population, Mattson (1990) conducted an investigation of developmental maturity and coping strategies in RN students. This exploratory descriptive study involved 138 students in one BSN completion program. Multiple regression and path analysis were utilized to analyze the data and resulted in two predictors of coping effectiveness: developmental maturity and past successful coping. While age and developmental maturity were not significantly related to coping, a strong link between developmental maturity and perceived coping effectiveness was found. Effective copers employed coping strategies which could solve the problem. Encouragement of problem-solving skills and use of support systems for ventilating feelings was recommended by the investigators to assist RN students deal with the stressors of continuing their education. This study was significant in that it also identified that older, re-entry women adjusted easier to their academic environment than younger students.

Motivational dimensions. Motivational factors of RNs for returning to the education arena were the focus of several investigations (Fotos, 1987; Lethbridge, 1989; Thurber, 1988; Lang, 1986). Fotos (1987) surveyed 57 RN students to identify reasons, or motivational dimensions, that precipitate returning to college. A modified Education Participation Scale (EPS) and a personal data form were used to assess the reasons for returning to school. Findings confirmed that nurses enrolled were primarily motivated just by a "desire for professional advancement" (p. 121). Pressures by society and personal reasons were of less importance. Fotos' interesting demographic results showed that a high percentage of registered nurses are working many hours and going to school either part time or full time, have expenses, children, and household responsibilities. The small sample size indicates a lack of basis to generalize. However, Fotos did show that orientation programs for new RNs are essential to provide information necessary for the RN to survive in school and that flexibility should be considered for this nontraditional student. Future studies could identify working conditions and responsibilities that impact upon quality of programming for these students.

Similar to Fotos, Lethbridge (1989) studied the motivational orientation (dimensions) underlying the reasons for RNs in rural New England to return to school. Lethbridge became interested in these reasons because of the limited financial rewards in rural areas for RNs to attain a baccalaureate degree and the great personal and financial hardship associated with returning to school. As a descriptive correlational study that identified the dimensions and underlying reasons subjects returned to school, the sample consisted of 132 RN students. The Educational Participation Scale, as modified by Carmody (1982), was utilized for data collection. Findings showed that three motivational factors were related to the decision to return to school: professional advancement, knowledge, and improvement in social welfare skills. In comparison to Carmody's (1982) previous study on urban nurses, Lethbridge's findings differed. Rather than professional advancement, Carmody found that knowledge was the first factor and improvement in social welfare skills was the second. No statistical comparison of Lethbridge's and Carmody's findings were possible because, while items loading on the factors were similar in content, they were not identical.

Thurber (1988) studied perceptions of nursing programs and attitudes toward professional nursing behaviors of 233 registered nurses upon entrance to and exit from two types of program (generic and second-step baccalaureate completion). Analysis of data collected from multiple sites identified factors motivating the student to return to school. Findings indicated that motivating factors for returning to school were enjoyment of learning by study (87.6%) and career advancement (88%). Two-thirds of the sample said they needed to improve job performance. Program choice results indicated 38.2 percent of the students entered generic RN programs and 61.8 percent entered second-step programs. Significant differences in program expectations were found at entry into the two types of programs, however, exit perceptions were more alike between students from these programs. The student profile of RNs enrolled in second-step programs revealed more males and younger, single Catholic women with fewer children than in generic programs. RNs in generic programs tended to be older, married women with greater family responsibilities and greater spouse support.

The findings of these studies suggest that registered nurses are not passive or submissive and that they cope with stress through social networking. Therefore, support of family, friends, and peers are significant factors for RN students. There is a need to further examine the learning motivations of the RN in the community. This should be a tremendous concern to educators. Future research should center upon examination of motivational dimensions within large RN populations and refinement of an instrument to assess these dimensions in the RN returning to school.

Curricular and Programatic Issues

The third general category of research focused on the development, comparison, and evaluation of the various types of programs and curricula offered to RNs returning for a baccalaureate degree in nursing. Seven studies focused on topics such as type of program and the program's impact, alternative types of programs, and placement policies (Arlton & Miller, 1987; Beeman, 1988; Blatchley & Stephen, 1985; Borst & Walker, 1986; Cragg, 1991; Lee, 1987; Tiffany & Burson, 1986).

Another area of interest is innovative teaching/learning strategies pertinent for the unique needs of the RN student. Microcounseling/interpersonal skills (Daniels, Denny, & Andrew, 1988; Farley & Baker, 1987), critical thinking (Sullivan, 1987), and locus of control (DuFault, 1985) were the focus of research investigations on strategies for teaching the RN student.

Types of programs. Lee (1987) examined stressful clinical and didactic experiences of the registered nurse returning to school. In this study, Lee identified and ranked stressful clinical and didactic experiences of 111 RN students, classifying stressful clinical incidents into "eight subcategories: patient care; assignment to a specific agency, service, or unit; relations with the staff; relations with the instructor or peers; evaluation of clinical performance; schedules; pressure to function as a registered nurse; and inadequate instructors" (p. 376). The highest mean scores for stress in the clinical setting were reported for scheduling, inadequate instruction, and relations with staff. Didactic incidents were classified into six subcategories: examinations and grades; inadequate instruction; relationships with instructors or peers; pressures of schedules; recitations; and papers. Lee found that papers, recitations, and relationships with instructors or peers evoked the most stress in the classroom setting. In comparing the stresses of clinical and didactic experience, didactic stressful experiences were more frequently reported than clinical experiences. In comparing registered nurse students enrolled in specifically designed RN/BSN programs with registered nurses enrolled in generic programs, registered nurses in the specifically designed programs identified inadequate instruction as the principle didactic area for stress. Those in generic programs identified examinations (specifically grades and schedule pressures) as the predominant stressor. Lee felt the major stress associated with learning for RNs was inadequate instruction. Consideration should be given to alternative modes of instruction. Implications for faculty include the need to be alert to situations that precipitate stress in the classroom and clinical setting so students can be assisted in achieving their goals.

Blatchley and Stephen (1985) investigated how the RN student fit into generic programs. They studied 57 National League for

Nursing approved generic programs which were randomly selected and asked specific questions related to admission policies for RNs, basic nursing credits required, special courses required, and the process of RN socialization. Results showed that admission requirements to university or college programs were fairly standard, including required test scores, transcripts, and challenge credits. Thirty schools required a GPA range from 2.0 to 2.7 with 2.5 the most common. Most schools required prerequisite credits to be met prior to admission. The number of basic nursing credits that could be earned by challenge varied from 14 to 47 with a mean of 30. The types of examinations utilized varied from national examinations, such as ACT-PEP, to teacher-made examinations. Seventeen schools developed special bridge courses for RNs to assist transition from technical to professional status. These schools felt the bridge course was the major process through which socialization occurred. A major concern in generalizing these findings was the small number of schools participating in the study.

In a national survey, Arlton and Miller (1987) identified advanced placement policies for awarding nursing and general education credit to RN students. A descriptive design was utilized to identify types of programs, specific types of credits awarded, nursing challenge programs, and general education support course challenges in 328 programs. Results showed that the majority of the programs (85%) were generic baccalaureate that admitted RNs while only 15 percent (N = 49) were RN only. Three-fourths (N = 238) of the generic programs indicated that 25 percent of their enrollment consisted of RN students, and 34 schools reported a 25–50 percent RN enrollment. The number of credit hours required in the RN-only programs ranged from 60 to 69, whereas in the generic programs, generally there are between 40–69 credit hours.

In awarding academic nursing credit, 95 percent of all schools provided the opportunity for RN students to obtain academic credit prior to the nursing major. Results showed that associate degree nurses were allowed to transfer credit from one academic institution to another, but diploma RNs were required to take some form of challenge examination. The most frequent type of examination used in generic programs were teacher-prepared (70%), and for RN programs ACT-PEP exams (53%). The range of number of courses that could be challenged varied among programs, with the majority of programs allowing approximately half of the nursing major to be challenged. The most frequently used clinical challenges were the NLN and ACT-PEP exams, and care plan preparation when enrolled in a course. Actual clinical examinations were required by 19 percent of the generic and 4 percent of the RN only programs. Many programs were generous with their challenge policies, but prohibited challenge in specific content areas such as research 58 percent, leadership management 47 percent, professional practice 47 percent, community health 37 percent, and advanced practice 36 percent. Programs reported using other challenge mechanisms for general education and support credit awards from 32 percent for sociology to 8 percent for anatomy and physiology. This study validated an increase in enrollment of RN students seeking programs that give recognition for past learning. The study identified that most programs allow challenging of courses and that most programs do not have a clinical challenge requirement. However, as Arlton and Miller (1987) indicated, most programs required teacher-made challenge examinations, and only half of the faculty reported having taken a college level course in test development. Given the lack of test development knowledge among faculty, the validity and reliability of these tests should be examined, and noted that while faculty offer great assistance for students to take nursing challenges, little assistance is provided for students to take general education challenge examinations. Future considerations for research should be given to these areas within baccalaureate programs.

In a descriptive comparative study, Beeman (1988) examined if there were significant differences between RN and generic baccalaureate students in their perceptions of their academic programs. Subjects included 284 undergraduate students from 12 programs, with 188 RN students (N = 59, in generic BSN programs; N = 129, in RN/BSN only programs) and 96 non-Rn students. The Beeman Educational Environment Measure for Adult Nurses was used to assess perceptions of their baccalaureate program, with reliabilities of the six subscales ranging from .65 to .92. Results showed that RN students in basic programs felt that some areas of their program inhibited learning. RN students in RN/BSN only programs felt their program promoted learning better, fostered self-direction/learning, and that practicality was enhanced. Qualitative data indicated RN students' need for greater flexibility in scheduling, more credit for previous experiences, and different requirements for entry. Several studies indicated that credit earned by challenge was a program option (Arlton & Miller, 1988; Blatchley & Stephen, 1985). In this study,

Beeman verified that RNs returning to school have different perceptions in their programs, and identified the importance of the structure of the educational environment to promote development. Strengths of this study include the large sample size and multiple data collection sites.

Although extension sites for RN/BSN programs have become prominent since 1978, little data is available on development and implementation of programming at these sites. The development of extension sites is increasing and should be more specifically researched. In one study, which addressed the above-mentioned need, Tiffany and Burson (1986) examined how extension sites were implemented by baccalaureate programs in 30 schools. These investigators identified three innovative curriculum models: the first model shifted instruction sites depending upon where most of the students lived; the second model had "outreach sites in a 700-mile radius with a single faculty member traveling to each site; and the third model modularized the courses and allowed independent study for courses.

Cragg (1991) assessed professional resocialization in a qualitative study of 24 RN students who had taken distance courses in nursing. Because distance education provided limited contact with faculty from the main campus, it was predicted that professional socialization would be less effective from a distance. Subjective reports were collected by telephone interview from students of four universities, with responses analyzed to determine whether professional socialization occurred and whether there was a difference between the group-oriented and the individual approach. Results showed that all students knew about professional issues, and attitudes and values expressed were congruent with professional organization. Differences identified in the schools were not based upon method of instruction but on the personality of the professor and/or personal attitudes of the instructor. Distance education is a growing method of providing access to a baccalaureate degree and a much needed area for research.

Borst and Walker (1986) evaluated the outcomes of one locally-based RN/BSN program, in a semiurban area 70 miles away from the parent institution. Outcomes of interest were whether or not there would be an increase in program enrollment: (1) if the program provided a needed service; (2) if there would be a positive student growth in skills and attitudes; (3) if graduation resulted in increased salaries and status for the RNs, and (4) if the graduates would achieve a higher level of personal satisfaction in education

and lifestyle. Study findings included an increase in program enrollment along with a description of the program's service to the
profession. Based on data from 16 graduates, 9 reported an increase in salary after completion of the program, 8 received pro-
motions in their place of employment, and 13 reported increased
self-esteem.

There is a need to increase accessibility of BSN nursing programs for RNs, especially in rural areas. Although the number of
off-campus sites has increased dramatically since 1978, little data
is available on the development, implementation, and effectiveness
of these programs.

Innovative teaching/learning strategies. There are many
areas in which innovative teaching/learning strategies should be
investigated. Published research regarding the development of
innovative strategies for teaching RN students has been very limited. Nursing education research studies identified teaching/
learning strategies related to such diverse topics as empathy, locus
of control, and improvement of interpersonal skills and critical
thinking skills.

Daniels, Denny, and Andrews (1988) conducted a study of empathy in relation to therapeutic communication skills of 53 RN
nursing students. An experimental design was used to assess the
degree to which nursing students acquired and retained communication skills taught through using a microcounseling technique.
Microcounseling was identified as a psychoeducational approach
that employs a highly systematic and structured method for teaching communication and interviewing skills. Subjects were randomly assigned to the experimental group which received
microcounseling, or to a nonattention control group. The treatment was 25 hours of microcounseling in basic communication.
Subjects were pre-tested and post-tested with the Carkhuff Indices
of Communication. Utilizing a multivariate analysis of covariance,
findings indicated that microcounseling significantly improved
empathy, reflection of feeling, and summarizing in the experimental group. Those who were taught using this approach made
less communication errors and asked fewer closed questions.
While particular study strengths include use of an experimental
design with random assignment of students to groups, the small
sample size limits the generalizability of the results.

Farly and Baker (1987) conducted a study focused on learning
interpersonal skills. This study examined the effect of selected,

self-management procedure training on the generalization and maintenance of interpersonal skills in a group of 24 registered nurse students. The students were randomly assigned to an experimental and control group. Both groups of students attended a workshop on interpersonal skills; in addition, the experimental group received training in specific self-management procedures, including post-workshop practice, self-monitoring, self-assessment, and self-reinforcement. Results showed that, on post-testing three months after the workshop, both groups maintained their knowledge of interpersonal skills equally well; however, on a measure of skill level in applying interpersonal skills, the experimental group performed significantly better ($p < .01$) than the control group. Caution should be observed in the interpretation of the findings because of the small sample size. However, the consideration that new behaviors could be learned through short-term training workshops and maintained over time could be significant for a variety of programs.

Rotter (1966) has described the concept of locus of control as either "internal," when the learner sees his other behavior affecting events, or "external," when events occur because of surrounding forces. It has been postulated that professional nurses should have an internal locus of control because the following professionally desirable characteristics are found to be related: a positive self-esteem, a sense of social responsibility, a hard working nature, a tendency for being achievement oriented, and an ability to problem solve.

DuFault (1985) investigated the characteristic of locus of control of registered nurse students. The purpose of this research was to determine if a course where exploration of the transition into a futuristic-oriented professional nursing role would move registered nurse students in a baccalaureate program toward stronger internality. A pretest-intervention-posttest experimental design was used to identify the effectiveness of a course titled "Transition into a Futuristic Professional Nurse." The sample consisted of 32 students in the experimental group and 32 students in the control group. The Rotter I-E Scale was administered as a pretest, posttest measure of personality construct of internal and external locus of control. A one-credit semester course, which focused on values clarification and commitment to the future of nursing practice, was the intervention for the experimental group. The students in the control group did not attend the classes. Change in the score from the pretest to the posttest was the criterion by which the experiment was evaluated. Results between the pretest, posttest areas indicated that the experimental group gained a significant difference in internality ($p < .0001$). A major study weakness concerns the sample population, which was not randomly selected, and thus lacking in adequate controls.

Sullivan (1987) examined if critical thinking, creativity, and clinical performance improved during a student's nursing program if the student's academic performance increased. Specifically, Sullivan studied the relationships between critical thinking, creativity, and clinical performance during the beginning and end of the student's program of study. Fifty-one registered nurses participated in the study. The instruments used to assess the three noted dimensions were the Watson-Glaser Critical Thinking Appraisal, Torrence Test of Creative Thinking, and the Steward Evaluation of Nursing Scale. Data were gathered upon entry to and exit from the program. Findings indicated that creativity scores at graduation were higher in flexibility but lower in originality. Clinical performance scores were found to be significantly higher at graduation with overall creativity scores being lower at graduation compared to entry into the program. Critical thinking skills showed no difference between entry and exit to the program. These results have implications for curricula development. Unfortunately, this study had a small sample size limited to one institution and inadequate controls.

DISCUSSION AND SUGGESTIONS FOR FUTURE RESEARCH

The areas of investigation and knowledge generated by the studies found in the published research over the past five years concerning RN student education indicates research efforts that have been fragmented and nongeneralizable. There have been few attempts to replicate previous research or to build upon existing research in the area. The theoretical frameworks utilized were based upon limited research in the areas of study. There were no prevalent theoretical models used across all studies and few acknowledged attempts were made to test theory. Most of the studies conducted tended to be descriptive in nature, using quantitative analysis with limited use of qualitative data. The major emphasis of current research has centered on describing the RN student currently enrolled in baccalaureate programs, and comparisons of differences between RN students and generic baccalaureate students on a variety of factors. Personal characteristics and program issues related to the registered nurse returning to school predominate the research literature on registered nurse students.

Other general concerns regarding the current research are that most studies were based on small sample size and used samples of convenience. A few studies attempted to use more than one site for data collection, however, only one study using an experimental design included subjects from multiple-data collection sites. In the studies reviewed, there was little indication of control for investigator bias, a concern in education research where the investigator commonly has some degree of investment in the educational processes under investigation. Many of the studies were related to program evaluation at a single site.

Strategies for data collection and measurement varied in the identified studies. Instruments tended to be well described and previously established reliability and validity were usually identified. No commonality of instruments were utilized under similar categories across the studies. The descriptive surveys often utilized researcher-made questionnaires or tests without reported psychometric properties or pilot study results.

As the profession of nursing moves toward greater autonomy and independence, educational programs must enhance learning experiences for the student so that autonomy and independence are rewarded rather than discouraged. In relation to content and categories, measurement of professional role orientation outcomes appeared to be a vital concern for nursing programs. Multiple roles held by adult female learners, benefits, and the involved costs were investigated. Future considerations need to include identification of these same issues for males, since they are becoming a larger part of the nursing student population.

A major category of study was student characteristics and needs, particularly since the RN student population's average age is increasing. There continues to be research related to the differences of the generic versus the registered nurse students in the areas of life stage, characteristics, and ego development. Furthermore, locus of control appears to be a factor that can impact upon the graduates' professional capability. In the future, research on curricular issues for this diverse population should be addressed, with consideration given to personal and academic factors affecting progression. Didactic and clinical instruction should be evaluated as well as desired outcomes at the professional level. Curricula can be redesigned based upon results of the research on RN students and programs.

Program comparisons between RNs and generic students and special programs for RNs continue to be identified in research studies over the past several years. Programs for RNs and generic students were found to differ in many areas. Differences were identified in program requirements and admission standards for RNs. Extension, or off-campus, sites for RNs were studied, which could be indicative of a growing need and response. Advanced placement, advisement, and recruitment of RN students have become major concerns of research.

Although the RN population is increasing in baccalaureate programs, a major concern is the relative lack of systematic research on this population within the last five years. With this student population increasing in size in every major college, research is needed to facilitate the RNs' level of education, assisting them with the multiple problems and issues encountered. Research regarding this population can contribute significantly to the knowledge base in curricula design. However, this can only be done if research on this population is valued. A variety of factors influence the choices nurse faculty make concerning the areas of research that faculty pursue. There is concern that there appears to be less research focused on nursing education, including this area of nursing education.

In conclusion, research studies concerning the registered nurse student are timely primarily because of the increased number of RNs who are returning to educational settings, and because of the unique characteristics of these students. It is imperative that nurse researchers increase the base of educational research related to this population.

REFERENCES

Arlton, D. M., & Miller, M. E. (1987). RN to BSN: Advanced placement policies. *Nurse Educator, 12*(6), 11–14.

Baj, P. (1985). Demographic characteristics of RN and generic students: Implications for curriculum. *Journal of Nursing Education, 24,* 230–236.

Beeman, P. (1988). RNs' perceptions of their baccalaureate programs: Meeting their adult learning needs. *Journal of Nursing Education, 27,* 364–370.

Bem, S. (1981). *Bem sex role inventory professional manual.* Palo Alto, CA: Consulting Psychologist Press.

Blatchley, M. E., & Stephan, E. (1985). RN students in generic programs: What do we do with them? *Journal of Nursing Education, 24,* 306–308.

Borst, B. B., & Walker, W. J. (1986). A locally-based baccalaureate nursing program for registered nurses. *Journal of Nursing Education, 25,* 168–169.

Campaniello, J. (1988). When professional nurses return to school: A study of role conflict and well-being in multiple-role women. *Journal of Professional Nursing, 4,* 136–140.

Carmody, C. E. (1982). *Motivational orientations of registered nurse baccalaureate students.* (Doctoral dissertation, Columbia University).

Cragg, C. (1991). Professional resocialization of post-RN baccalaureate students by distance education. *Journal of Nursing Education, 30,* 256–260.

Daniels, T. G., Denny, A., & Andrews, D. (1988). Using microcounseling to teach RN nursing students skills of therapeutic communication. *Journal of Nursing Education, 27,* 246–252.

DuFault, M. (1985). Changing locus of control of registered nurse students with a futuristic-oriented course. *Journal of Nursing Education, 24,* 314–319.

Dugas, B. W. (1985, May). Baccalaureate for entry to practice: A challenge that universities must meet. *The Canadian Nurse,* 17–19.

Everett, H. (1988). Personality characteristic of registered nurses in baccalaureate education. *Nurse Educator, 13*(5), 27–36.

Farley, R., & Baker, A. J. (1987). Training on selected self-management techniques and the generalization and maintenance of interpersonal skills for registered nurse students. *Journal of Nursing Education, 26,* 99–102.

Fotos, J. C. (1987). Characteristics of RN students continuing their education in a BS program. *The Journal of Continuing Education in Nursing, 18,* 118–122.

Gunter, L. (1969). The developing nursing student, Part III: A study of self-appraisals and concerns reported during the sophomore year. *Nursing Research, 18,* 237–243.

Heinemann, E. (1964). The conflicting life of a student. *Nursing Outlook, 112,* 35–38.

King, J. (1986). A comparative study of adult developmental patterns of RNs and generic students in a baccalaureate nursing program. *Journal of Nursing Education, 25,* 366–371.

King, I. (1988). Differences between RN and generic students and the impact on the educational process. *Journal of Nursing Education, 27,* 131–135.

Kolb, D. (1974). *Building a learning community.* Washington, DC: National Training and Development Service Press.

Lange, L. L. (1986). Recruiting, advising, and program planning for RN/BSN students. *Western Journal of Nursing Research, 8,* 414–430.

Lawler, T., & Rose, M. (1987). Professionalization: A comparison among generic baccalaureate, ADN and RN/BSN nurses. *Nurse Educator, 12*(3), 19–22.

Lazarus, R. (1966). *Psychological stress and the coping process.* New York: McGraw-Hill.

Lazarus, R. (1976). *Patterns of adjustment.* New York: McGraw-Hill.

Lee, J. (1988). Analysis of coping methods by returning RNs. *Journal of Nursing Education, 27,* 309–313.

Lee, J. (1987). Analysis of stressful clinical and didactic incidents reported by returning registered nurses. *Journal of Nursing Education, 26,* 372–379.

Lethbridge, D. J. (1989). Motivational orientations of registered nurse baccalaureate students in rural New England. *Journal of Nursing Education, 28,* 203–209.

Levinson, D. (1978). *The seasons of a man's life.* New York: Ballentine Books.

Linares, A. Z. (1989). A comparative study of learning characteristics of RN and generic students. *Journal of Nursing Education, 28,* 354–360.

Loevinger, J., & Wessler, R. (1970). *Measuring ego development: Construction and use of a sentence completion test.* San Francisco: Jossey-Bass.

Lubno, M. (1984). *Cost effectiveness analysis of selected baccalaureate and associate degree nursing education programs in Texas.*

Unpublished doctoral dissertation, The University of Texas at Austin.

Lynn, M., McCain, N., and Boss, B. (1989). Socialization of RN to BSN. *Image, 21,* 232–237.

Mattson, S. (1990). Coping and developmental maturity of RN baccalaureate students. *Western Journal of Nursing Research, 12,* 514–524.

MacLean, T. B., Knoll, G. H., & Kinney, C. K. (1985). The evolution of a baccalaureate program for registered nurses. *Journal of Nursing education, 24,* 53–57.

NLN, 1991. *Nursing data review.* New York: National League for Nursing Press.

Radloff, L. (1977). The CES-D scale: A self-report depression scale for research in the general population. *Applied Psychological Measurement, 1,* 385–401.

Rendon, D. (1988). The registered nurse student: A role congruence perspective. *Journal of Nursing Education, 27,* 172–177.

Rotter J. B. (1966). Generalized expectancy for internal versus external control of reinforcement. *Psychology Monographs, 80,* (No. 609).

Stember, M. L. (1984). Curricular research in nursing. In Werley, H.H. & Fitzpatrick, J.J. (Eds.), *Annual review of nursing research, Volume 2.* New York: Springer.

Sullivan, E. (1987). Critical thinking, creativity, clinical performance, and achievement in RN students. *Nurse Educator, 12,* 12–16.

Swanson, M. J. (1987). Baccalaureate nursing education: Students' perceptions of roles, effort, and performance. *Journal of Nursing Education, 26,* 380–383.

Thurber, F. (1988). A comparison of RN students in two types of baccalaureate completion programs. *Journal of Nursing Education, 27,* 266–273.

Tiffany, J. C., & Burson, J. Z. (1986). Baccalaureate nursing education at extension sites: A survey. *Journal of Nursing Education, 25,* 124–126.

USDHHS (1988). Secretary's Commission on Nursing, Final Report Volume I. Washington, DC: USDHHS.

Weathersby, R. (1977). A developmental perspective on adult's use of formal education (Doctoral dissertation. Howard University).

Dissertation Abstracts International, 38A.7085-A-7086A (University microfilms No. 7808621).

Wolfe, D., & Kolb, D. (1979). Career development, personal growth and experimental learning. In D. Kolb, I. Rubin & J. McIntyre (Eds.), *Organizational psychology: A book of readings* (3rd ed.). Englewood Cliffs: Prentice-Hall, Inc.

Chapter Five

A REVIEW OF LITERATURE ON CHANGING ANSWERS ON MULTIPLE-CHOICE EXAMINATIONS

Patricia A. Haase, RN, MSN

Carol P. Riley, RN, DSN

Linda Dunn, RN, DSN

Susan Gaskins, RN, DSN

To change or not to change . . . how are nursing students being advised? Nurse educators must become aware of the research findings related to changing answers on multiple-choice examination. Students and faculty generally believe that it is better not to change initial answers on multiple-choice examinations (Benjamin, Cavell, & Shallenberger, 1984). Many faculty and test-taking skill books still advise students to stick with first impressions, go with intuition, and "your first answer is probably the correct answer" (Kussler, 1988, p. 190). This advice has persisted in spite of mounting research to the contrary.

Student learning is assessed in many schools of nursing by multiple-choice examinations. Considering the fact that, ultimately, graduates of nursing schools must pass a multiple-choice licensing examination in order to practice within the nursing profession, it is imperative that nursing students develop sound test-taking skills.

What is the belief of the students and faculty with reference to changing answers on multiple-choice examinations? What characteristics of the student or the test would affect the outcome of changing answers? The purpose of this review of literature is to examine the research on changing answers on multiple-choice examinations in relation to faculty and student beliefs, student characteristics, and test characteristics.

METHODOLOGY

Twenty-two research articles (see Table 1) were reviewed, only two of which were found in the nursing literature. All studies

Table 1.

First Author	Year	Sample Size	Discipline	Percent of Changes Rate	R/H	H/H	H/R	Statistical Methods	Other Variables
Best	1979	261	Psychology	3.75	21	17	62	chi square	item difficulty
Cassidy	1987	56	Nursing	3.1	16	13	71	chi square	feedback
Foote	1972	384	Psychology	7.7	22	24	55	% frequency	item difficulty, test anxiety
Green	1981	70	Statistics		1.63*	1.36*	4.09*	ANOVA	item difficulty, beliefs
Jacobs	1972	44	Education		20	24	56	ANOVA	
Jordan	1990	284	Nursing	6.07	18	26	55	chi square	level of class
Matter	1986		Elementary Education		17	27	56	MANOVA	race, income
McMorris	1987	120	Education	6.4	1.5*	1.2*	3.7*	t test	reasons/changing, item difficulty
McMorris	1986	51	Education	6.9	1.7*	1.2*	5.4*	correlation	item difficulty, intervention
Mueller	1975	471	Education	3.7	17	18	65	correlation	impulsivity, gender, anxiety
Payne	1984	296	Elementary Education	6.27	24	22	54	2 × 2 factorial MANOVA	test anxiety, race, and gender
Penfield	1980	83	Statistics					Hilcoxon Matched Pairs	gender and rank in class
Ramsey	1987	95	Statistics	6.6				Fisher's LSD ANOVA	item difficulty, confidence
Reiling	1972	416	Education	9				multiple regression	cognitive, grades, item difficulty
Schartz	1991	104	Education	7.4	26	18	56	ANOVA, correlation	reasons/changing, strategy, gender
Shatz	1987	65	Psychology	4.4	20	25	55	correlation	reasons/changing
Sitton	1980	65	Psychology	6.6	1.68*	0.89*	4.14*	Pearson R	personality
Skinner	1983	68	Psychology	4.03	26	22	52		gender
Slem	1985	470	Psychology	4	0.48*	0.48*	0.87*	t test	instruction
Smith	1979	157	Psychology	6	26	12	62	ANOVA	gender, rank in class
Torrence	1986	100	Adult Ed	8.36				chi square	different population
Vider	1980	162	Education	3.6	1.45*	2.0*	4.91*	correlation	item difficulty

*Reported as statistical means, R/H = right to wrong, H/H = wrong to wrong, H/R = wrong to right. All other numbers are percentages.

reviewed consistently demonstrated that changing answers resulted in more changes from wrong to right and in higher test scores. These findings were true regardless of other variables studied in relation to changing answers. Changes made from wrong to right (W/R) ranged from 52 percent (Skinner, 1983) to 71 percent (Cassidy, 1987), while changes from right to wrong (R/W) ranged from 16 percent (Cassidy, 1987) to 26 percent (Skinner, 1983; Smith, White, & Coop, 1979), and wrong to wrong (W/W) answer changes ranged from 13 percent (Cassidy, 1987) to 27 percent (Matter, 1986).

Faculty and Student Beliefs

Faculty beliefs. Only one study focused on faculty beliefs concerning changing answers. Benjamin, Cavell, and Shallenberger (1984) conducted a survey of 58 faculty members at a Texas university. Fifty-five percent of the faculty believed that changing initial answers on multiple-choice examinations would lower scores, 16 percent believed that scores would improve, 10 percent believed scores would remain neutral, and 19 percent didn't know. Of this group, 63 percent usually warned their students not to change their initial answers. None of the instructors who believed that changing answers would improve scores passed this advice on to their students.

Student beliefs. Generally, from the review of literature, students did not believe that changing answers would improve their score. Yet, in spite of this belief, they changed answers. The methodologies used to discover student beliefs on changing answers were varied. Mueller and Shwedel (1975) and Smith, White, and Coop (1979) reported student beliefs about answer changing, but did not discuss the method in which they obtained this information. Mueller and Shwedel (1975) found that 64 percent of their educational students believed that changing answers would result in a lower score while 36 percent believed that the score would neither be raised nor lowered. None of the subjects in this sample believed that their score would be raised. Smith, White, and Coop (1979) reported that although 86 percent of the students changed their answers, only 7 percent believed changing would result in a higher score, 68 percent believed that they would decrease their score, and 25 percent felt it would make no difference in their final score.

Foote and Belinky (1972) administered a show of hands survey on 384 students and found that the subjects were equally divided into thirds. One third believed that changing answers would result in a lowered score, one third thought their score would be increased, and one third thought their score would remain unchanged. The purpose of the study was to provide feedback regarding the consequences of answer-changing behavior and to measure the end result and rate of changes on two subsequent examinations. Even though the students were informed that 57 percent of their changes on previous examinations had resulted in a change from W/R, neither the level of success nor the rate of change were altered in the subsequent examinations.

Jacobs (1972) assessed student beliefs regarding changing answers by asking 44 subjects to write a brief note about their opinion on answer changing and expected results. He obtained similar results to Foote and Belinky's (1972) study in that there was no relationship between perceived expectation of the student and actual gains.

In a sample of 68 psychology students, Skinner (1975) obtained student beliefs using a 24-item student information survey. The folk admonition against changing answers was found to be prevalent and he attributed the low rate of 4.03 percent of changing answers to this belief. The researcher postulated that if students felt negative towards changing answers, students would not make a change unless there was high probability that the changed answer would be correct. Thus, the high rates of gain in earlier studies were due to a reluctance on the part of the students to change their answers. In this study, 52 percent of the changes were W/R. The conclusion was that answers should not be changed unless the probability of gain was high.

In order to study the effects of intervention on students beliefs and answer-changing behavior, Slem (1985) randomized 471 students into an intervention group and a non-intervention control group. Both groups were pre- and post-tested with the intervention group receiving lecture and discussion on the answer-changing myth and strategies under which to change answers. Results showed no significant differences in rate of change between the groups. The author concluded that there is a discrepancy in answer-changing beliefs and behavior. Even though students in the non-intervention group believed it was not beneficial to change answers, they did so anyway.

McMorris was the primary investigator (McMorris, DeMers, & Schwartz, 1987; McMorris & Weideman, 1986) in two research studies to discover why students changed their answers despite their beliefs that such action would result in a loss. Earlier research had consistently reported high gains that were attributed to reluctance of the students to change answers unless there was a high degree of confidence the changed answer would be correct. The researchers proposed that instructing students of the benefits of changing answers would cause them to change more answers and some of the gains would evaporate. The researchers did not pre-test or survey the students for previously held beliefs. The two groups were presented with the results of previous research indicating the benefits of changing answers. The graduate students in both research studies then were given examinations and a questionnaire containing a 7-point scale measuring attitudes toward changing answers and were asked to choose a reason why they changed their initial answer. Students were limited to five researcher-chosen reasons for changing answers: making a clerical error, finding a clue in the item, rethinking and conceptualizing a better answer, rereading and understanding the question better, and learning from a later item. A favorable attitude was found toward changing answers. Reasons for changing answers were rethinking and reconceptualizing a better answer (57 percent), rereading and better understanding (28 percent), clerical error (8 percent), finding a clue (3 percent), and learning from a later item (3 percent). Correlations of answer-changing behavior with attitude towards changing, reasons for changing, and test anxiety were not significant. The instructed sample was compared to uninstructed samples of similar graduate classes. These comparison groups were called "patched-up control groups" (McMorris & Weideman, 1986, p. 98). No differences were found in the rate of change or amount of gain, negating the alternate hypothesis that previous high gains were caused by reluctance of students to change answers.

The studies cited indicated that there is no relationship between student beliefs, faculty beliefs, and actual behavior on multiple choice examinations. In each study, the percentage of changes made and the number of correct changes made remained constant. As a result, Slem (1985) concluded that intervention and resources to enhance performance were unnecessary and could be spent in other ways, while others suggested appropriate instructions should always be given to the students regarding the benefits of changing initial answers (McMorris & Weideman, 1986; Smith, White, & Coop, 1979).

STUDENT CHARACTERISTICS

Several different student characteristics were examined in relation to answer-changing behavior. The student characteristics examined in the 22 reviewed articles were: population, gender, personality, test anxiety, level in class, strategies, confidence, and guessing.

Populations

In the 22 articles reviewed, the sample population consisted mostly of college students in psychology or education (see Table 1). Two studies included nursing students (Cassidy, 1987; Jordan & Johnson, 1990); two studies included elementary children (Matter, 1986; Payne, 1984), and one study included adults who were taking their journeyman-level certification examination (Torrence, 1986). The findings of these studies consistently show the prevalence of W/R changes and net gains from changing answers, suggesting that these results may be generalizable to all students.

Gender

No relationship between different genders and net gain was found in 6 studies (Mueller & Schwedel, 1975; Payne, 1984; Penfield & Mercer, 1980; Reiling & Taylor, 1972; Schartz, McMorris, & DeMers, 1991; Sitton, Adams, & Anderson, 1980). In a relatively small sample (68) in which there was more than twice the number of females (n = 46), Skinner (1983) reported the only statistically significant gender difference, finding that females changed more answers than males and had less success. This finding was contrary to the general finding that more changes equal more success and to the numerous other studies that established no significant difference when comparing the different sexes. The small number of males (n = 22) in this sample may have contributed to the irregular findings.

Personality

Only one study attempted to correlate personality with students' patterns of changing answers. Sitton, Adams, and Anderson (1980) measured 65 students' personalities by using the Beck Depression Inventory, the Dominance Scale of the California

Psychological Inventory to measure assertiveness, the Taylor Manifest Anxiety Scale, and the Eysenck Personality Inventory to measure introversion-extroversion. From stepwise multiple regression analysis, the four best predictors for the number of changes were extroversion, assertiveness, course grade, and depression. The best predictors for improvement in score were being extroverted, being married, and being assertive. No similar studies or replications could be found to refute or substantiate these findings.

Test Anxiety

Test anxiety was another student variable that was investigated in relationship to answer-changing behavior. In a sample of 70 college students, Green (1981) administered a 25-item Test Anxiety Scale in addition to the multiple choice examinations. The findings supported the hypothesis that high test anxiety resulted in changing more answers than did low test anxiety. Both high and low test-anxious students profited proportionally. Payne (1984) investigated test anxiety in 296 eighth graders and did further analysis in relation to race and sex. Test anxiety was measured by a 15-item validated instrument called Survey of Feelings About Tests. Black and female students were found to have higher test anxiety scores. As found in Green's (1981) study, higher test anxiety correlated with more changes. However, blacks made more R/W changes which was not the expected direction. The mean score (71.21) for black students was considerably lower than the mean score (92.57) for white students, which the author concluded may have been a manifestation of high anxiety or lack of test-taking skills. Further research is recommended before a relationship between test anxiety and changing answers can be established.

Level in Class

Nine studies attempted to discover if there was a relationship between the student's level in the class and the net gains made from changing answers. Various methodologies and statistical methods were used. For example, to determine the level in the class, one study used single test scores (Ramsey, Ramsey, & Barnes, 1987) and one study (Reiling & Taylor, 1972) used the final grade in the course for their calculations. Best (1979) and Penfield (1980) divided their samples into thirds based on a single examination and

Penfield (1980) eliminated the middle third and compared only the high and low group. The remaining studies (Jordan & Johnson, 1990; Mueller & Schwedel, 1975; Schartz, McMorris, & DeMers, 1991; Shatz & Best, 1987; Smith, White, & Coop, 1979) used the results of more than one examination and divided the sample into thirds and compared the different groups.

The findings of these studies were inconsistent. Jordan and Johnson (1990) through analysis of the variance, found no significant differences in improvement of scores among the lower, middle, or upper thirds of the sample. Best (1979) used Chi Square Analysis and learned that the upper third level of the students did the least amount of answer changing and the middle and lower third were equal in their amount of changing. The upper and middle third make more W/R changes on difficult items whereas the lower third made more W/R changes on easy items. The lower third also made as many R/W changes on easy or difficult items. In contrast, Penfield (1980) using the nonparametric Wilcoxon Matched Pairs Signed Ranks Test, found that high-scoring students made more changes than the low-scoring students and high-scoring students made more W/W changes than the low. In Mueller and Schwedel's (1975) study, high-scoring students made fewer W/W changes. Mueller and Schwedel (1975) also found that the lower third did not experience net gains as large as the middle and high-scoring groups. Schartz, McMorris, and DeMers (1991) obtained similar results, but Reiling and Taylor (1972) found the opposite to be true with their low-scoring students making slightly better net gains from the changed answers. Smith, White, and Coop (1979) also found that low-scoring students made more gains, but may have obtained better results by calculating the scores on a prechange basis in order to eliminate the compounding effect of calculating gain scores after answer changing had improved the scores.

From these studies, no relationship between the level in class and net gain could be established. Generally, all levels continued to make gains from changing their answers, but no group consistently did better or worse than the others.

Strategies

Test-taking strategies in answer changing was explored in one study (Schartz, McMorris, & DeMers, 1991). From interviewing a sample of 104 students, six separate strategies emerged: leaves blanks and rereads unsures; leaves blanks and rereads all; answers all, marks unsures, and rereads unsures; answers all, marks unsures, and rereads all; answers all; answers all and rereads unsures; and answers all and rereads all. Due to the small sample, no test strategy was significantly different, but several patterns emerged. A majority of the students reread their items and the students who reread all the test items made more changes and made more gains. A curious finding of Schartz, McMorris, & DeMers, (1991) was that, as a test strategy, 70 percent of the students left blanks for initial responses. The researchers concluded that this phenomenon may mean that the percentage of answer changes reported in most of the previous studies on answer changing may have been underestimated.

Confidence

Because Skinner (1983) had concluded that answers should not be changed unless students had a high confidence level that the new answer would be correct, the focus on Ramsey, Ramsey, and Barnes' study (1987) was confidence level. In a sample of 95, students were asked to complete an answer-changing questionnaire following a multiple choice examination describing all changes, reasons for changing, and confidence level on a scale of 0 to 100 percent. Using a two-factor, independent groups analysis of the variance and testing pairwise difference with the Fisher's least significant difference (LSD) procedure, the researchers learned that most answer changes resulted in significantly greater gains regardless of how low or high the confidence level. However, the easier the item and the higher the confidence, the greater the gain.

Guessing

In another variable related to confidence, Shatz and Best (1987) reported that students who used guessing as a reason for changing answers were not nearly as likely to benefit from changing answers. With guessing, the percentage of W/R dropped to 35 percent. The student had almost an equal chance of changing answers from W/R (35 percent), W/W (34 percent), and R/W (31 percent). The researchers concluded that in testing situations, if a student is unsure of an answer, agonizing over alternatives is unproductive and a waste of time.

A serious limitation of this study was the small sample size (65). No other studies have been done on guessing; yet, Shatz and Best (1987) reported guessing to be the most common reason for changing answers. Guessing had not been given as an alternative on the questionnaire in the studies that dealt with reasons for changing (McMorris, DeMers, & Schartz, 1987; McMorris & Weideman, 1986). In the Schartz, McMorris, and DeMers' study (1991), questionnaires were not used and reasons for changing were given by interviews. While guessing was never mentioned as a reason for changing answers, two frequently cited reasons were "unsureness of the first answer" and "something just clicked" (p. 168).

TEST CHARACTERISTICS

Some of the researchers in the 22 reviewed articles attempted to explain or correlate differences in answer-changing behavior to test characteristics. The test characteristics most frequently examined were: cognitive level, item difficulty, and item discrimination.

Cognitive Level

Two studies looked at the cognitive level of items as a variable in changing answers. Reiling and Taylor (1972) tried to relate answer-changing behavior to items that required analytical reasoning. In a sample of 416, no significant difference in the rate of change or net gain was found in changing analytical questions versus non-analytical questions. A serious limitation of this study was the lack of criteria by which the questions were classified as analytical and the lack of such classification by independent judges.

Smith, White, and Coop (1979) attempted to rectify the limitation of Reiling and Taylor (1972) by classifying the cognitive level of items into two accepted levels: lower order items and higher level items. Lower level items tested knowledge or comprehension. Higher level items tested cognitive processes such as application, synthesis, analysis, or evaluation. The researchers hypothesized that greater gains would result from changing higher order items. Although more changes were made on higher level items, no difference was found in the proportion of gains to losses on lower level and higher level items.

Item Difficulty

The test characteristic most frequently examined in relation to answer-changing behavior was item difficulty. Item difficulty was usually defined as a p-value or a proportion of the students who answered the item correctly. This value had a different operational definition in each study. Jacobs (1972) used analysis from a pool of previous tests. His test contained equal numbers of easy (p = .75), moderate (p = .49), and difficult (p = .29) items. Best (1979) classified his items as easy or difficult based on whether the item fell above or below the median percentage of correct answers. McMorris and Weideman (1986) and McMorris, DeMers, and Schartz (1987) assigned item difficulty as the percent of test-takers answering an item correctly with a mean of 75 and 73 respectively. Green (1982) categorized items as easy (p = .70–1.0), moderate (p = .40–.69), and difficult (p = 0.0–.39) both pre- and post-answer changes. Ramsey, Ramsey, and Barnes (1987) used three slightly different p values: easy (.75–1.0), moderate (.51–.74) and difficult (0–.50). Vidler and Hansen (1980) did not discuss their methodology for classifying item difficulty.

A concern of some researchers was whether item difficulty values derived from the same data would be valid due to the compounding effects of answer changing. Jacobs (1972) bypassed this concern by using data compiled from a pool of previously taken tests. Green (1981) measured the item difficulty both before and after answer-changing and concluded that there was no significant difference in results. Best (1972) calculated that this possibility was remote—in order for one item to be altered from difficult to easy it would have to receive 9 to 10 times the mean number of W/R changes.

The results of the studies of item difficulty and answer-changing behavior varied. Jacobs (1972) found the greatest gains from changing answers were made in the low to moderately difficult items. Vidler and Hansen (1980) found the opposite to be true. This result may have occurred because the test used in their study was the Watson-Glaser Critical Thinking Appraisal, which tested a student's ability to think at different levels. McMorris and Weideman (1986) found students made more changes in the difficult items, but there was no significant difference in the amount of gain. In the study of Ramsey, Ramsey, and Barnes (1987), the mean gain for easy items was significantly greater that the mean gain for difficult items. Jacobs (1972) found the least amount of changes with the easy items and the least amount of gain with the difficult items. Green (1981) found that difficult items elicited the most changes with the least amount of gain. McMorris, DeMers, and Schartz (1987) got similar results and discovered that more W/W changes were made on difficult items.

Item Discrimination

Item discrimination was sometimes discussed in conjunction with item difficulty. The operational definition of item discrimination in studies by McMorris, DeMers, and Schartz (1987) and McMorris and Weideman (1986) was the proportion of the top third of the class answering the item correctly minus the proportion of the bottom third of the class. Greater item difficulty and item discrimination were positively correlated with more frequent changes and negatively correlated with gain scores (McMorris, DeMers, & Schartz, 1987).

The research by McMorris, DeMers, and Schartz (1987) was the only replication study that dealt with test characteristics. Because of the varying operational definitions and methodologies used, no definite conclusions can be generalized. Two trends that emerged were difficult items are changed more often and more gains are made on easy items.

CONCLUSIONS AND RECOMMENDATIONS

A review of the published research on changing answers on multiple-choice examinations indicates that it is beneficial for students to change answers. While the research in nursing was limited to two studies, both supported the previous research that has been done in other disciplines. Nursing students need to be advised that judicious answer changing on multiple-choice examinations is recommended.

Several limitations were noted in the studies reviewed. Many of the studies utilized a small and/or convenient sample. All the studies failed to describe a conceptual framework to guide the research endeavor. Only a minimal number of studies had been replicated.

This review of literature has addressed changing answers on paper and pencil multiple-choice exams. As early as 1994, the format for the NCLEX-RN exam may change to Computer-Adaptive Testing (CAT) and candidates for registered nurse licensure will no longer take a paper and pencil exam. Most forms of computerized testing do not allow review of previous questions or answer changing once the enter key of the computer has been pressed. Methods of assisting students to develop appropriate test-taking strategies for computerized testing need to be explored.

Further research efforts are needed to identify other variables that affect the behavior of changing answers. Examining personal attributes, decision-making characteristics, and the reading level of students are areas that could provide insight into the behavior and result of changing answers on multiple-choice examinations.

REFERENCES

Benjamin, L. R., Cavell, T. A., & Shallenberger, W. R. (1984). Staying with initial answers on objective tests: Is it a myth? *Teaching of Psychology, 11,* 133–141.

Best, J. B. (1979). Item difficulty and answer changing. *Teaching of Psychology, 6,* 228–230.

Cassidy, V. (1987). Response changing and student achievement on objective tests. *Journal of Nursing Education, 26*(2), 60–62.

Foote, R., & Belinky, C. (1972). It pays to switch? Consequences of changing answers on multiple-choice examinations. *Psychological Reports, 31,* 667–673.

Green, K. (1981). Item-response changes on multiple-choice tests as a function of test anxiety. *Journal of Experimental Education, 49,* 225–228.

Jacobs, S. (1972). Answer changing of objective tests: Some implications for test validity. *Educational and Psychological Measurement, 32,* 1039–1044.

Jordan, L., & Johnson, D. (1990). The relationship between changing answers and performance on multiple-choice nursing examinations. *Journal of Nursing Education, 29,* 337–340.

Kusler, D. (1988). Teaching students how to take an examination. *Journal of Emergency Nursing, 14,* 190–191.

Matter, M. K. (1986). *Eenie, meenie, minie, mo —change this answer— yes or no?* (Report No. TM 860682). San Francisco, CA: Annual Meeting of the National Council on Measurement in Education. (ERIC Document Reproduction Service No. ED 276 739)

McMorris, R. F., DeMers, L. P., & Schwartz, S. P. (1987). Attitudes, behaviors, and reasons for changing responses following answer-changing instruction. *Journal of Educational Measurement, 24,* 131–143.

McMorris, R. F., & Weideman, A. H. (1986). Answer changing after instruction on answer changing. *Measurement and Evaluation in Counseling and Development, 19,* 93–101.

Mueller, D., & Shwedel, L. (1975). Some correlates of net gain resultant from answer changing of objective achievement test items. *Journal of Education Measurement, 12,* 251–254.

Mueller, D., & Wasser, V. (1977). Implications of changing answers on objective test items. *Journal of Educational Measurement, 14,* 9–13.

Payne, B. D. (1984). The relationship of test anxiety and answer-changing behavior: An analysis by race and sex. *Measurement and Evaluation in Guidance, 16,* 205–210.

Penfield, D. A., & Mercer, M. (1980). Answer changing and statistics. *Educational Research Quarterly, 5,* 50–57.

Ramsey, P. H., Ramsey, P. P., & Barnes, M. J. (1987). Effects of student confidence and item difficulty on test score gains due to answer changing. *Teaching of Psychology, 14,* 206–210.

Reiling, E., & Taylor, R. (1972). A new approach to the problem of changing initial responses to multiple choice questions. *Journal of Educational Measurement, 9,* 67–70.

Schartz, S. P., McMorris, R. F., & DeMers, L. P. (1991). Reasons for changing answers: An evaluation using personal interviews. *Journal of Educational Measurement, 28,* 163–171.

Shatz, M. A. & Best, J. B. (1987). Students's reasons for changing answers on objective tests. *Teaching of Psychology, 14,* 241–242.

Sitton, L. R., Adams, I. G., & Anderson, H. N. (1980). Personality correlates of students' patterns of changing answers on multiple-choice tests. *Psychological Reports, 47,* 655–660.

Skinner, N. F. (1983). Switching answers on multiple-choice questions: Shrewdness or shibboleth? *Teaching of Psychology, 10,* 220–222.

Slem, C. M. (1985). *The effects of an education intervention on answer-changing behavior.* (Report No. CG 018875). Los Angeles, CA: Annual Convention of the American Psychological

Association. (ERIC Document Reproduction Service No. ED 266 395)

Smith, M., White, K. P., & Coop, R. H. (1979). The effect of item type on the consequences of changing answers on multiple-choice tests. *Journal of Educational Measurement, 16,* 203–208.

Torrence, D. R. (1986). *Changing answers as a testing strategy for taking objective tests.* (Report No. TM 870336). Kansas City, MO: Annual Meeting of the American Evaluation Association. (ERIC Document Reproduction service NO. ED 282 920)

Vidler, D., & Hansen, R. (1980). Answer changing on multiple-choice tests. *Journal of Experimental Education, 49*(1), 18–20.

DATE DUE

HIGHSMITH 45-220